A Hospital Handbook
on Multiculturalism
and Religion

A Hospital Handbook on Multiculturalism and Religion

Revised Edition

Neville A. Kirkwood

MOREHOUSE PUBLISHING

First published in 1993 by Millennium Books,
an imprint of E.J. Dwyer (Australia) Pty. Ltd.

Morehouse Publishing, 4775 Linglestown Road, Harrisburg, PA 17112
Morehouse Publishing, 445 Fifth Avenue, New York, NY 10016
Morehouse Publishing is an imprint of Church Publishing Incorporated.

Cover design by Dana Jackson

Library of Congress Cataloging-in-Publication Data

Kirkwood, Neville A.
    A hospital handbook on multiculturalism and religion / Neville A. Kirkwood. –Rev.
ed.
        p. cm.
    Includes bibliographical references (p.129)
    ISBN 10 0-8192-2184-8 (pbk.)
    ISBN 13 978-0-8192-2184-1
1. Hospital patients –Religious life. 2. Minorities—Hospital care. 3. Medicine—
Religious aspects. 4. Multiculturalism. I. Title
RA965.6.K57 2005
362.11'088—dc22   2004023715

Printed in the United States of America

16   8 7 6 5

⇢ CONTENTS ⇠

✢ ACKNOWLEDGMENTS ✢

THE FOLLOWING ORGANIZATIONS ARE HEREBY acknowledged for their helpful responses to my inquiries
and for their publications:

The Maronite Church (Sydney diocese)
The Syrian Orthodox Church of Antioch
The Greek Orthodox Archdiocese of Australia
The Church of Christ Theological College,
    Sydney
The Salvation Army
The Seventh-Day Adventist Church
The Roman Catholic Church (Sydney
    archdiocese)
The Baptist Union of N.S.W.
The Anglican Church (Sydney archdiocese)
The Church of Jesus Christ of Latter-day Saints
The National Spiritual Assembly of the Baha'is
The Lothian Community Relations Council,
    Edinburgh

The Australian Buddhist Vihara Institute
The Buddhist Council of N.S.W
The Presbyterian Church of Australia
The Islamic Council of N.S.W.
The N.S.W. Jewish Board of Deputies
The Lisa Sainsbury Foundation, London
The Hospital Chaplaincies Council, London
Ms. Pamela Bennet, Japan
Nursing Times, Macmillan Publishing, London
The Evergreen Taoist Church of Australia

✦ FOREWORD ✦

Australia is now the most multicultural nation in the world. This diversity of peoples of different cultures and religions offers an important challenge for health services committed to a provision of care that is not only appropriate and accessible but recognizes and values people's different cultural and religious backgrounds.

An individual's culture and religion form fundamental parts of his or her makeup and are particularly important when that person is seriously ill and in hospital. It is recognized that different cultural behaviors and religious beliefs can lead to misunderstandings between health professionals and the people in their care. It is therefore important for staff to be sensitive to the particular attitudes and needs of their patients and of the relatives of those patients.

Reverend Dr. Kirkwood's hospital handbook represents a commendable effort to provide accessible information on this diverse and complex topic and is a valuable addition to our growing knowledge about the needs of our multicultural society. It provides insight into the different beliefs and practices of the major religions, as well as discusses the significance of certain religious attitudes and rites to the lives of the people of these religions. It also includes information on what action may be taken by laypersons in some emergency situations, action that may bring comfort and peace of mind to those concerned.

I believe that if used to complement information gained directly from patients and professionals it will prove most useful for the continuing development of appropriate and sensitive health care for people here and elsewhere.

B. J. AMOS
Director-General
N.S.W. Department of Health
Sydney, Australia

✦ INTRODUCTION ✦
TO THE REVISED EDITION

The first edition's reception and interest has been maintained for more than a decade. East Asians are to be seen in increasing numbers around the world as professionals, traders and students. The omission in the first edition of Chinese religions was major. The practice of *Tai Chi* in many Western societies as a form of relaxation and stress relief has made many aware of Taoism. In this edition, Taoism and Confucianism are considered along with Jainism of Indian origin. Additions to provide a clearer understanding have been made in other sections.

The present disturbed state of international relations makes it important that all of us should have some understanding however slight of the beliefs and practices of our neighbors. Never has there been a time when world peace has been under so much threat. Every effort to make ourselves more aware of how our neighbors around the world understand and view life will make us more accepting of them and them of us.

In health-care institutions we can play our part in promoting international harmony and goodwill as well as providing more acceptable care.

✦ INTRODUCTION ✦

Many health-care workers, including chaplains, are unfamiliar with multicultural needs and requirements. This handbook is intended to be a ready-reference for those who work in hospitals and similar institutions dealing with the sick.

The last half of the twentieth century saw distance become of minimal consequences in our world. The movement of people from country to country either as tourists, refugees or in migration has escalated in recent decades.

It started with the population shifts following World War II. Independence from colonial powers saw many nationals of their former colonies taking advantage of concessions granted by the former rulers. And there was also the resettlement of postwar displaced people from Europe.

More recently the wars in Indochina and the Middle East, particularly Lebanon, have resulted in the considerable resettlement of the victims of those wars. Indochina, with its many differing cultures, has added new dimensions to Australia's multicultural mix. The Middle East situation has enabled it to be more widely recognized here where previously it was comparatively unknown.

The developing of the economies of Korea, Hong Kong and Japan has spread their people abroad. Their appearance in Western society (either as migrants, businesspeople or tourists) means that they are being met in our hospitals and health-care institutions. As the Japanese culture involves an intermingling of practices, there is a final chapter, "Japanese Beliefs and Practices," to enhance understanding in this area.

As I said at the beginning, this book is intended for reference. However, in any country where cultures intermingle, the practices of a particular culture, which include its religious aspects, are likely to be modified or adapted to the parameters of the local environment. Thus this is a handbook providing guidelines that should not be used as a substitute for or to avoid face-to-face assessment of the patient's own religious views and practices. Rather it should be used, as Dr. Amos suggests in his foreword, to supplement information coming directly from the patient and family and only used as the first source of information where this information is not directly available from the patient or family themselves.

ONE

A Multicultural Society

The debate over multiculturalism and integration or assimilation has been—and sometimes still is—a minefield of insensitivity on both sides. Host cultures are often intolerant of the differences that peoples of other cultures bring. The newcomers expect their host to permit them to live and function as they would in their native land. Differences in the standard and style of living are often ignored.

A move from a third-world country to the West brings such a contrast that sometimes the adjustment is made even more difficult. A need to maintain cultural practices is necessary for the stability of the newcomer in a strange land. The desire to live close to fellow countrymen, which establishes cultural enclaves, is natural. Yet this very process is often misunderstood. People grieving for a homeland need support both from fellow countrymen and from the citizens of their adopted country.

The one area where all must be treated on equal terms is in the health-care field. Health-care workers have a reputation for being caring, understanding people. Because of this, they are aware that these newcomers have different beliefs and customs that need to be considered in the hospital setting. Different religious traditions have led to certain practices and behavior. These need to be respected, particularly when and where a person is dying. Respect for these requirements is essential for the healthy grief of the relatives and friends. The staff also need to be comfortable in the knowledge that what they have done is acceptable.

It is easy for our Western psychology–trained hospital bereavement counselor to be alarmed, for instance, that members of a certain group of a particular ethnic origin are apparently showing no sign of grief or are not talking about the imminent death of their family patriarch. It may be the practice in these people's culture for the second-degree male relatives (e.g., uncles or cousins) to be the ones with whom the doctors and staff discuss the nature of the patient's diagnosis and response to treatment. The second-degree relatives then decide who and how much should be told. Often the nuclear family of the relative is unaware of the seriousness of the illness.

People from such a background fear to mention the possibility of a terminal condition. For them to name a condition is to open the possibility for its fulfillment. Social workers, chaplains, nurses or doctors who raise the question of possible death, without first endeavoring to understand the cultural stance, are likely to bewilder and confuse the family. There may even be a communication breakdown between the medical team and the patient's kin.

To assume that because patients are in a Western hospital they can shed millennia of cultural inheritance to conform with different cultural perspectives is to misunderstand the value of cultural practice. For some it may adversely affect the progress or response to treatment. It is not a clear-cut case of either assimilation or multiculturalism. There needs to be a marriage of the two. The staff and patient each must seek to learn from each other, each being prepared to not only live as neighbors but also to respect areas of habit or cultural emphases in the interests of harmonious cooperation.

Within health-care institutions socioreligious concerns are of great importance, no matter the country of origin or religion of the people involved. Of course, there are always some who are devout in their religious practice and others who are indifferent.

Due deference should be given to the socioreligious requirements of hospital patients, particularly in a time of crisis. Offers of assistance to seek out the appropriate religious person for the patient must in no way give the appearance of interfering with or embarrassing the patient. The priest of the patient's faith should be notified.

In hospitals where there are numbers of patients of different ethnic backgrounds, staff should make some effort to be aware of these differences. In each religion there are groups with different emphases or differing sects or denominations, as found within the Christian religion. It is not possible for each health-care worker to be able to identify all these divisions. With a sense of caring, the particular persuasion or preference of the patient may be ascertained either from the patient or the relatives.

There may be members of staff who belong to the same faith, whether they are domestic, catering or ward staff. If a professional interpreter is not available a staff member may be requested to ascertain the religious position of the patient and identify the patient's significant advisor, priest, imam or rabbi. There may be other appropriate ways of discovering the desired information, but if there are language problems, using an experienced interpreter is the ideal solution.

It cannot be overemphasized that not only may people from other backgrounds have practices and beliefs that differ from Western Christianity, but it also must be understood that religious traditions are part of culture. The culture of an Asian Christian may therefore differ from the cultural practices of a Greek or Dutch Christian. There are cultural distinctions as well as specifically religious variations to daily living: a Vietnamese Christian, for instance, will have customs and beliefs that will differ from those of a Vietnamese Buddhist. Similarly a Vietnamese Christian will have needs that may not be entirely akin to an Australian-born Christian's requirements; and, further, a Roman Catholic patient will desire certain sacraments to be administered while a Baptist may not be so insistent, though all are Christians.

When it comes to hospital bedside treatment and procedures during hospitalization or death, the staff should consider certain questions as far as possible. These involve diet, fasting, names, symbols, birth and handling of the body on death. Some of these basic matters will be outlined in the following pages.

Integration or Westernization to varying degrees depends upon the patient's age and education; some allegiance to cultural roots must be expected. The health-care worker must be alert to discern to what degree the ways of the country of adoption have been absorbed by the patient and family members. This can vary from person to person and within a family. The patriarch or matriarch of a family may be the key to the amount of assimilation that has taken place. He or she may be so revered as to be able to enforce within the family the strict observance of cultural traditions.

On the other hand, for example, a Hindu patient who in his own country was a strict vegetarian may readily eat meat, even beef, in his new land.

Assessing the needs of each patient and family shows how strictly they observe their culture and religion. This may be done at the initial admission by a questionnaire that includes matters of diet, religious persons to contact and fasting or other specific needs, such as special arrangements when using the toilet. (Many people from the East prefer water cleansing rather than the use of toilet paper.)

The following chapters, which deal with each religion or culture separately, should be used as background information and as a guide. They should not be used as a substitute for the opportunity to talk with a patient or family about their religion and culture. Sincere inquiries about their beliefs and practices break down fears and worry about being misunderstood. Your interest opens the way for mutual appreciation and cooperation within the ward. This in turn makes for a patient who is more ready to accept the necessary treatment and hospitalization in a strange environment.

→ TWO ←

Christianity

In the Western world, Christianity has dominated history, religion, politics, law and education for centuries. In the last half of the twentieth century humanism, secularism, materialism, more recently the "new age" movement and the influence of Marxism and neo-Marxism have seen a decline in the awareness and practice of Christianity. Basic biblical knowledge, its meaning and application are not as widespread nor are the practices of the various denominations of the Christian church, some of which have undergone reform, so well-known. In looking at Christians' needs we shall consider them under five major groupings, noting any particular variation in practice. They are Catholics, Orthodox, established churches, nonconformists and others, a more or less historical division.

Catholics: Roman, Maronite, Jacobite, Melchite and Ukrainian.

Orthodox: Eastern (Russian and Greek), Syrian, Serbian, Coptic, Armenian, Lebanese, Bulgarian, Polish and Macedonian.

Established churches (i.e., those churches that were recognized and established as the church of the state): Anglican (Church of England, Episcopal), Lutheran, Church of Scotland, Reformed Dutch.

Nonconformist, Independent (those churches that separated from the established churches): Baptist, Church of Christ, Congregational, Methodist, Presbyterian, Salvation Army, Seventh-day Adventist, Uniting Church, Pentecostal and neo-Pentecostal.

Others: Church of Jesus Christ of Latter-day Saints (Mormons), Jehovah's Witnesses.

The Catholic, Orthodox and some established churches have an episcopal form of church government, that is, a system of bishops. They place a stronger emphasis on the position and status of the clergy. Generally the priest's principal ministry is the administration of the sacraments. For many of their parishioners who are patients in a hospital, receiving the sacraments is important in a religious sense, as well as having therapeutic benefit.

For nonconformists and some others, the ministry of the sacraments plays an important but less central role in worship and the life of the church. The ministry of the word, biblical teaching and pastoral care (other than the sacramental) have the greater emphasis.

Christians believe that Jesus, born about 6 BCE in Bethlehem in Judea, was the messiah, or Christ, promised during the previous millennia to the world through the Hebrews by their God, Yahweh. This messiah was to be God in human form. This Jesus is God from eternity. The death experienced by Jesus is the means of atonement whereby men and women may experience the forgiveness of God and be restored into a personal relationship with him. True Christianity is not knowledge or belief in a set of historical events; rather it is the acceptance of those historical events as God acting to draw humankind to himself in unique intimacy. It is a spiritual communion between God and the believer. Through this relationship, God's way of love and peace is demonstrated to the historical world.

Christian pastoral care in the hospital setting is carried out in the name of Christ. The integrity of the Christian carer may be sufficient testimony of the Christian nature of the care offered. At other times it is appropriate for the counselor to share the Christian way in the course of the caring or to provide Christian spiritual support and comfort through Scripture reading, sacrament, prayer and other means.

RITUALS AND SACRAMENTS

Most religions have set rituals and sacraments. Christian denominations variously celebrate the major events in a person's life such as birth, marriage and death. There are also other sacraments that hold spiritual significance, such as confession (reconciliation), anointings and the Eucharist (holy communion) that may be important for many hospitalized people.

Catholic Group

A visit from a chaplain or parish priest is considered normal practice. Such a visit will ascertain the patient's need for the sacraments. Any request for a chaplain or priest should be treated as of utmost importance. Catholics believe the spiritual needs should be given higher priority than the physical and temporal.

The chaplain or priests are able to provide more than sacramental ministry; giving counsel and emotional support are roles that they willingly accept with the patients or relatives.

Baptism

This sacrament brings to a person a share in the life of Christ and membership in his church.

When a baby or unbaptized Catholic person's life is in danger, the chaplain or priest should be called. In an emergency, if a chaplain or priest is not available, any person may baptize. In such cases the baptizing person pours water on the child and says the words: "I baptize you in the name of the Father and of the Son and of the Holy Spirit." When an emergency baptism is conferred, the chaplain or priest is to be notified later, so that details may be registered.

Reconciliation (confession)

This sacrament brings to the Catholic in a particular way a loving God's reassurance. The sacrament can be given only by a priest. Privacy is essential.

Holy communion

Catholics believe that Jesus is present in this special sacrament and therefore the communicant is united with Christ in a special way. The sacrament of holy communion may be administered by a priest or a person who has the endorsement of the chaplain. The chaplain or priest will consult staff in deciding whether Holy Communion can be given to a patient (who may be nauseated or fasting before an anesthetic) who may have requested it. Where necessary, patients can be given a particle so small that it will not interfere with medical or surgical procedures.

Anointing of the sick

In this sacrament patients are offered the compassion of Jesus for the sick; it gives them strength and peace. It is given only by a priest. A patient may be anointed more than once during the same illness. Catholics have an expectation that a priest will be called in a case of emergency and this should be done when a known Catholic lapses into unconsciousness or is unable to communicate his or her wishes. This sacrament is not given to a person who has died; therefore a chaplain or priest should be called before death occurs.

A sacramental ministry by a Roman Catholic priest is acceptable to patients of the other Catholic churches identified here when a priest of their own church is unavailable.

Orthodox Group

Baptism

If a newborn babe's condition warrants serious concern for its survival, a priest should be contacted, with the parent's consent, for the sacrament of holy baptism.

If an Orthodox priest is not available, any Christian priest or minister may perform an emergency baptism by raising the child in the air and saying: "The servant of God (name) is baptized in the name of the Father and of the Son and of the Holy Spirit. Amen." If lifting of the child is not possible, then baptism may be administered by placing the right hand on the bowl of water that should be available. The Orthodox priest should be informed of such emergency baptisms.

Confession

When requested by the patient, the priest should be called. Privacy for total confidentiality should of course be provided if possible.

Holy communion

This may be received as often as possible for spiritual and bodily sanctification. Patients scheduled for an operation should receive holy communion the day before if possible. Holy communion given at such time is not equivalent to last rites. Baptism precludes the necessity for last rites for the Greek Orthodox patient.

Last anointing

The Syrian Orthodox priest administers the sacrament of the last anointing. Usually it is administered before death, but may be dispensed after the patient's apparent death in the hope that the Spirit is still in the body. Prior to this anointing, confession and holy communion should be offered if possible.

Established Group

Baptism

In an emergency, a staff member such as a nurse may pour a little water on the baby's head saying: "(Name), I baptize you in the name of the Father and of the Son and of the Holy Spirit." When there is time, the chaplain or clergyperson should be called. The one officiating would desire (if possible) to meet the parents before conducting the baptism. Certificates of baptism should be issued. If the baby survives, the parents should contact the parish minister to complete the service.

Holy communion

This is celebrated by a fully ordained clergyperson or licensed layperson. Communion is usually provided on the request of the patient or relatives. It is desirable, when possible, that more than one person with the minister celebrate holy communion.

Last anointing

Many Anglican dioceses practice a last anointing of the dying. Prayers and other offers of comfort and support are given by the church to the family at the time of death, on the request of relatives.

Nonconformist or Independent

The Salvation Army does not observe any of the sacraments, such as baptism or holy communion.

Baptism

Baptist, Church of Christ, Seventh-day Adventist, and some Pentecostal and neo-Pentecostal followers practice believers' baptism. This service is conducted only after the individual has reached an age where an understanding of a personal faith in Christ is possible. The other churches in this group, like the previous groups, baptize infants (although some individual ministers also recognize believers' baptisms). In emergencies, the requirements are similar to other churches who baptize newly born babies whose lives are threatened. There is less emphasis upon the need for the baptism of a dying child. The parent's desires and beliefs should be honored.

Infant dedication or presentation

Those who do not baptize infants have an infant dedication or presentation service. Where the parents request such a service at the bedside in an emergency, the appropriate chaplain or minister should be called. The short service includes Bible readings and prayer appropriate for the occasion.

Holy communion

These churches regularly celebrate services of holy communion. The patient may request. Communion, and the chaplain or minister available is able to accede to the request.

Anointing of the sick

This is practiced with varying degrees of acceptance and regularity. There is a growing practice of a healing ministry through anointing. It is almost invariably performed at the request of the patient. The chaplain or minister, with elders or deacons present, conducts the anointing.

The Order of St. Luke, which has supporters from most denominations including Catholic, established and free churches, holds a balanced stance on anointing and healing of the sick. Representatives may be called in by relatives for anointing and prayers of healing. The pentecostal and neocharismatic churches strongly hold to a position of faith healing. Caution should be exercised with people who see illness as demonic and stress the need for "deliverance" through exorcism.

Last anointing

There are no last rites. The chaplain or minister prefers to be called to be with the patients and relatives before death takes place. The chaplain or minister considers it a privileged ministry at the bedside of the one dying, to be with the relatives, offering prayer, comfort and support.

Others

Church of Jesus Christ of Latter-day Saints (Mormons): If the patient requires a sacrament, the state president or church leader will provide the sacrament each Sunday upon notification.

Jehovah's Witnesses do not celebrate sacraments such as baptism, anointing or holy communion. On each eve of Jewish Passover they celebrate the death of Christ in a eucharistic type of service. This is their only sacramental form of service.

DIET AND FASTING

Catholics

Usually Catholics are required to fast as preparation for holy communion; as a penance; during the season of Lent; or as any other worthy spiritual exercise or form of devotion.

These are not always observed by Catholics these days.

Some may make special efforts during Lent, which are looked upon as a self-denial. They may abstain from eating meat on the first day of Lent and all the Fridays of Lent. Patients may inform hospital staff of any such special devotions. However, most would not insist upon following these in the hospital.

Where medical and therapeutic reasons suggest otherwise, the Catholic is not obliged to conform to the usual church regulations in regard to these matters of fasting and abstinence. (In fact, the patient may be conscience-bound not to follow the regulations in order to aid the healing process.)

Orthodox

A seriously ill patient may be excused from following dietary obligations during Lent. During this period an Orthodox person is expected to abstain from meat and all animal products, e.g., milk, cheese, butter, eggs.

Established and Nonconformist Churches

Generally there are no obligatory dieting restrictions. However, some may personally practice abstinence and fasting. Seventh-Day Adventists ban the use of tobacco and alcohol; the use of tea and coffee is discouraged. For them a modified vegetarian diet, which includes dairy products such as milk, butter, cheese and eggs, is recommended. The eating of flesh is discouraged and the consumption of scripturally forbidden food is not permitted. The practice of vegetarianism is widely varied and is regarded as a health matter rather than religious regulation. The dietary desires of an Adventist should be something that staff ascertain on admission.

Others

The Church of Jesus Christ of Latter-day Saints (Mormons) follow a dietary code that carries the weight of a commandment. Alcohol, tea, coffee, tobacco and cola drinks are to be avoided; although they are not vegetarians, they are encouraged to eat meat sparingly.

CARE OF THE ILL AND DYING

All Christian denominations desire the offer of pastoral and spiritual care to their hospitalized parishioners. The local minister or priest will endeavor to make contact with known church members or may use lay pastoral care people to follow the patient's stay in the hospital. It is during the period prior to death that the sacramental ministries of baptism, reconciliation (confession) and anointing should be administered. Where the sacrament of anointing is practiced, it may be administered several times.

Sacramental ministry, as indicated earlier, has highest priority in the Catholic and Orthodox churches. Established churches also offer their members holy communion during their hospital stay. The other churches and the Mormons offer the Lord's Supper (communion) upon request.

In the Western world, hospital procedures are based generally on Christian practice. Generally there are no special procedural requirements necessary following death. Most ministers or priests would prefer to be called to see the patient and meet the family prior to the death so that more effective care of the family after death may be offered.

All churches would emphasize the dignity of the human body, alive or dead. Each body should be handled with the greatest care respecting this dignity. Normal hospital procedures for handling the body after death are acceptable to all Christian churches.

AUTOPSIES, TRANSFUSIONS, TRANSPLANTS

Considering always the emphasis upon the dignity of the body, there are no religious objections to the conducting of an autopsy or the administering of blood transfusions or to the donation or receipt of organs for transplantation.

An important exception is the Jehovah's Witnesses, however, who are opposed to blood transfusions. A Witness receiving a transfusion will be excommunicated.

When a Catholic patient has any doubt or question of conscience in any of these matters it ought to be discussed with a Catholic priest. The priest has necessary competence to advise, inform or guide the person who is faced with such difficulties.

As a basic principle, with a few exceptions, Christian churches leave decisions on these matters to the individual conscience of the professional and the patient.

ABORTION AND FAMILY PLANNING

Here we find the churches at variance in their belief and practice. Most believe that human life begins at conception and that interference with the normal development raises moral, ethical and legal issues of considerable weight and that any decision on abortion should not be made without due consideration of these.

Catholic Group

In general the Catholic church rejects the following on moral grounds: Abortion—no matter how early it is; abortifacient procedures, drugs, etc.; the contraceptive pill, creams, devices (IUDs); tubal ligation; vasectomy or any other form or method of sterilization.

The church recognizes the so-called natural family planning method, which is built upon the ovulation cycle. "With this method it is possible for a couple to avoid the 'contraceptive' mentality. . . . Rather it encourages a spirit of responsible parenthood which a couple can use right from the first day of their marriage together." Thus responsible parenthood was advanced and advocated by Pope Paul VI in his encyclical *Humanae Vitae* (1968).

Where medical circumstances raise the question of need for the termination of a pregnancy, a Catholic couple may seek a consultation with a Catholic priest to enable a decision in good faith and with a peaceful conscience.

Orthodox Group

The Syrian Orthodox church considers abortion in all its forms to be wrong—"simply murder." A pregnant woman should not consent to an operation that threatens the life of a child without consulting a priest.

The Greek Orthodox position is similar in prohibiting any medical procedure that would terminate the life of the fetus or embryo. However, in case of hemorrhage, procedures designed to stop the bleeding as distinct from procedures for expelling the living attached fetus are permissible, even if fetal death eventuates.

Established, Nonconforming and Other Groups

These churches stand for the sacredness of human life. The moral and ethical dilemmas in this area are understood. "Abortion on demand" would not be officially condoned. A termination of pregnancy is mostly acceptable if, for medical reasons, the mother's life is in danger. As a form of birth control it is unacceptable. The mother or couple's right to make a judgment with a clear conscience is often the accepted procedure after a sincere consideration of the ethical issues involved in the case.

The advance of modern medical knowledge and technology raises the ethical problems in such matters as surrogate motherhood, artificial insemination by a donor and in vitro fertilization. These have left the churches in a position where they cannot offer definitive answers in theology.

Each circumstance must be considered in its uniqueness and left to the individual conscience. These churches generally have no problems with the use of contraceptives and other procedures in birth control and family planning.

MODESTY

All the denominations of the Christian church recognize the sacredness and dignity of the human body and accept the need for the treatment of that body with modesty. This sense of modesty will vary from individual to individual and from generation to generation. Some female patients might prefer to be cared for by a female doctor and nurse, but these days, health care professionals are able to meet the needs of all patients without embarrassment. Where agitation on the grounds of modesty is shown or expressed, staff should be allocated accordingly, if possible, showing due respect.

→ THREE ←

Islam

The word *Allah* is the Arabic word for God. Muslims, Christians and Jews worship the one God. The roots of the three religions go back to the time before Abraham, who is the common link.

Islam means "submission" or "the act of submitting oneself"; *Muslim,* from the same root, carries the meaning "one who submits." Therefore a Muslim is one who submits to Allah.

A follower of Islam is not a Mohammed-an, but a Muslim. The use of the former term or any type of equivalent is likely to offend.

Mohammed (peace be upon him), the founder of Islam, was born 570 CE at Mecca. At age forty he went into a desert cave to meditate. In the last days of the month of Ramadan he received a vi-sion. This and later revelations became the basis of the Qur'an, or Koran. Nonacceptance of his teaching caused his flight to Medina in 622 CE Later that year, 300 of his followers defeated an army of 1,000 men. Thus *jihad*, or holy war, began. In 630 CE with 10,000 armed men he captured Mecca. Thus the Islamic faith was established. He died in 632 CE and is believed to be the final prophet.

Mohammed (peace be upon him) prescribed a special way of life and rules known as the Five Pillars of Islam:

Confession of Faith daily in front of witnesses—
   "There is no God but Allah and Mohammed is his prophet."
Prayer five times a day facing Mecca and with prescribed washing, ritual and gestures.
Fasting during the month of Ramadan: For twenty-eight days no healthy Muslim may eat, drink or smoke between dawn and sunset.
Almsgiving, a sign of Islamic brotherhood.
Pilgrimage to Mecca, known as the *haj*.

The absolute singularity of Allah (monotheism) is the basis of the Muslim's concept of God. He is the creator, controller and governor of the universe. A believer's life and property belong to God. The fear of life, personal safety or pain demonstrates a lack of belief and submission to Allah. Everything that happens in a person's life has been determined by Allah within the first forty days of conception. Complaint against the vagaries of life is considered as criticism of Allah's will for the individual. (It is not uncommon for a Muslim to interrupt a sentence to say in Arabic "Praise be to Allah" or "Thanks be to Allah" [*hum'dullah*] every time there is a twinge of pain. This is to be seen as a gracious acceptance of the pain planned by Allah.)

As Allah is the controller of human lives, he is also the provider of all things necessary to fulfill his will in a person's life. Muslims therefore often do not show fear and doubt about their hospitalization.

Muslims are appalled at the permissive Western *Christian* society. They are continually warning their people not to lower their own moral standards in family matters, sexual looseness, alcohol consumption, dress, gambling, etc. Some Muslims who have become more integrated into Western society have moderated their living style, which is causing concern to Muslim leaders. These fears and concerns may be carried into the hospital. Such tensions are to be noted and assurances of respect for Islamic beliefs and practices indicated by staff.

DIET AND FASTING

The eating of pork, bacon, ham or any other by-product of pork is strictly forbidden, nor should these items come into contact with any other food that is to be eaten by Muslims. Alcohol is totally forbidden, even its use in small quantities in preparing meals, puddings or cakes.

Muslims are allowed to eat beef, mutton and poultry provided the meat is *halal* (killed and prepared by a Muslim according to Islamic law). There are no restrictions on fish, vegetables, dairy products and fruit.

Some Muslims may refuse to eat hospital food and may insist on having food brought into them. The older generation is usually very conservative. In cooperation with hospital staff, patients or their relatives may be consulted to ascertain any dietary preferences, as hospital food may prove unappetizing for Muslims, who often prefer spicy foods.

Ramadan is usually a month of fasting. Fasting is not required of the sick, the traveler and

nursing mothers. The two big Muslim festivals
are the *Eed-ul-Fitr*, which ends Ramadan, and
Eed-ul-Azha, which commences the *haj* (pilgrimage to Mecca). This *Eed* also commemorates
Abraham's willingness to offer his son as sacri-
fice. (The Muslim tradition identifies the son of
Ishmael, Hagar's son, and not Isaac, Sarah's
son.) The family may request that the patient be
given leave to go home for those two days. Like
Christmas cards, Eed cards are sent. Wishing the
patient a happy Eed by the staff is appreciated as
an expression of goodwill to Muslim patients.

Examinations, tests and surgery should be
avoided, if possible, on an Eed day.

PASTORAL AND SPIRITUAL CARE

In Islam it is mandatory for an imam or spiritual
leader to visit the sick in hospital if called. If
there is a request for an imam, mulvi or sheikh,
the request must be followed through. In practice
many imams are in secular employment and
carry out their duties as teachers at the Friday
mosque prayers. As their time is limited, they
may not be able to visit the patient in the hospital. The reciting of special portions of the Koran
under certain conditions is necessary. These may

be recited and prayers offered by relatives or friends. Any prayers offered by an imam are in Koranic form. They do not name the patient as this would be deemed a criticism of Allah's will for the patient.

Prayers from a Christian minister or official pastoral care person may be acceptable, as Jesus is the only healing prophet in the Qur'an.

AUTOPSIES, TRANSFUSIONS, TRANSPLANTS

Routine or nonessential autopsies are not permitted. Where it is necessary for the issue of a death certificate or for coronial purposes an autopsy is accepted. As a body is to be resurrected on the last day, it should be buried intact. Thus organ donations are not made generally. However, organ transplants may be received where medical need dictates. Blood transfusions are acceptable for Muslim patients.

RITUALS

Birth

No religious sacrament or ritual is required except that a member of the child's family recite a prayer in the baby's ear as soon as convenient after birth.

Arrangements should be made for the circumcision of a male child as soon as possible after the birth. Comments by hospital staff criticizing the practice are considered distasteful and unprofessional.

Ritual ablutions and washing

Muslims have strict rules for ritual washing hygiene practice.

Mosques provide adequate water for purification before prayers. Cleanliness for them is important. Preparation for worship, for instance, includes the washing three times of face, ears, forehead, feet to ankles, hands, arms to elbows, the sniffing of water up the nose and washing out the mouth. Wet hands are rubbed through the hair to remove dust. A devout Muslim may wish to do this five times a day, although exemption because of illness is possible.

In personal cleanliness showering is preferable to a bath. Toilets should be provided with a jug that can be filled with water as Muslims need to wash their private parts after urination or defecation. It is not possible to pray without this washing.

ABORTION AND
FAMILY PLANNING

Birth control would generally be considered an endeavor to circumvent Allah's will for life. Pressure to practice birth control should not be asserted, rather it should be explained. According to the degree of Westernization, devotion, education or economic circumstances, the need for birth control will be considered.

Abortion is forbidden unless the mother's physical and mental health are in danger.

CARE OF THE ILL AND DYING

A dying Muslim may desire to sit or lie facing Mecca. That is, northwest in Australia and to New Zealand; southwest in the United Kingdom and Europe; west to southwest in North America. The movement of the bed to such a position is deeply appreciated. Relatives may recite portions of the Koran around the bed. If there are no relatives, then any Muslim may offer such help and comfort.

As the patient is dying, a pillow should be put under the head to elevate it above the rest of the body. The Muslim call to prayer, the *Kalima,* should be recited by friends. *Sura* (chapter) 36 of the Qur'an is also appropriate. It ends "all glory to Him who controls all things! Unto Him you shall all return."

Even though there is an acceptance of and an acknowledged submission to Allah's plan for their life and his timing of their death, many Muslims are fearful when dying. Maybe it is a fear of their state in the future life. On which rung of the ladder of seven hells and seven heavens will they find themselves? Death is a taboo subject for Muslims.

Grief counseling is not well accepted. It may even be considered an intrusion of privacy. Dying patients may show passivity, which may be for one of three reasons: a resigned acceptance of their fate; disguised fear, since fear would indicate lack of trust in Allah's judgment and mercy; or guilt over inadequate submission prior to illness. They passively accept the perceived punishment for their sins of commission and omission.

Expressions of grief vary according to the age and sex of the dying patient. Slapping, scratching and punching the body as expressions of grief are encountered and condoned. They are, however, contrary to Muslim belief. To mar the body that Allah made affronts Allah.

Regarding euthanasia, Muslims would consider the stopping of medical procedures as a contravention of Allah's will for the patient's life. The timing of death is in Allah's hands.

Handling of the deceased body

Only Muslims if possible should handle the body in the hospital—a male for a male, a female for a female. If a Muslim is not available, then non-Muslims should use disposable gloves so as not to touch the body.

The eyes should be closed; the lower jaw should be bandaged to the head to stop a gaping mouth. The body is then straightened. The limbs and joints are first flexed several times before being placed in final position.

The body should not be washed, nor hair or nails cut; the body should be covered, the head turned right, to face Mecca when buried.

The body is removed by a funeral director authorized by the Islamic community, who will wash and prepare the body for burial according to Muslim procedures.

If there is any doubt, the local Muslim community should be consulted.

MODESTY

Nakedness is anathema to a Muslim and hospitalization does not lessen the sensitivity. Women usually are fully covered from head to foot, even in bed, so that their body form may not be seen. The requirement to don only a hospital gown for surgery or other reasons is likely to be met with opposition.

Some Muslim women may refuse an internal examination prior to birth.

Men always remain covered from waist to knee. Any less clothing even in front of other men is offensive.

Medical examinations of patients in front of a number of doctors and students of both sexes is objectionable.

This attitude can, of course, create problems for hospital staff. Male Muslims should be examined by men. Similarly only female nurses and doctors should examine Muslim women. More conservative Muslim males may have an objection to females being in charge of their medical or nursing care. They may object to the concept of a woman having a position over them about which they can do little.

Again, older devout males may wish to keep their head covered at all times. Staff should respect this desire, not making any fuss or reference to it.

A SIGNIFICANT CULTURAL DIFFERENCE

Many Muslim cultural groups have strict procedures concerning the discussion of medical information with family and patient. Second-degree male relatives of the patient, e.g., uncles and cousins, should be informed of any diagnoses, procedure and prognosis. They in turn consider the wisdom or otherwise of telling the patient and immediate family. Our Western society and medical practice find this objectionable as it runs counter to the civil rights of the patient. Some Muslims, however, prefer it to be this way. Patients then do not have to contemplate the future life at that stage and this enables them to proceed through the illness without the resigned acceptance of death or trying to disguise fear or guilt of judgment of past sins. Doctors and nursing staff would be wise to ascertain the family's desires in information sharing. Such acknowledgment is

likely to bring far greater cooperation and support of the medical team by the relatives. It
would be wise to lay some ground rules by iden-
tifying the persons to be told and limiting their
number to two or three.

→ FOUR ←

Judaism

The Jewish people have had a history of dispersions across the known world from 722 BCE e.g., Assyria, Babylon, Spain, Poland and Odessa (Ukraine). Some were affected by the cultures of their adopted countries. In many countries they were forced to live in ghettos and maintained strict solidarity. In others, although they retained their distinctiveness, a greater integration weakened their conservatism. There were, however, those who retained their rigid orthodox traditions. Even in modern Israel and elsewhere some are still strictly orthodox, wearing eighteenth-century dress and not cutting their hair. Others have adopted reformed and conservative positions. Conservative Jews hold a middle ground between orthodox rigidity and a reformed position that has discarded some Jewish rituals and attitudes. As a result of the post–70 CE dispersion, many Jews have adopted food habits, dress and codes of conduct of their adopted lands. However, each observes the Torah with varying degrees of literalism. Health-care workers should carefully ascertain to which group their patient is aligned. This is important as a Jewish patient's belief may vary from no belief in a life beyond death to a belief in full bodily resurrection and immortality of the spirit. Most Jews would accept the belief that the human spirit returns to God.

Judaism stresses human responsibility in this life and therefore is not fatalistic. A religious Jew places emphasis upon living a moral and ethical life rather than being preoccupied with eternal rewards. Judaism, from its earliest days, observed many rituals, several of which were rites of passage. The two main rites that do not concern life's stages are the Sabbath and the Passover.

Sabbath is from sunset on Friday evening to sunset Saturday evening or from the first sighting of three stars. Orthodox Jews strictly observe it as a day of rest. Attendance at synagogue, saying of prayers and the lighting of candles are all part of Sabbath worship. There are certain limitations as to what may or may not be done on the Sabbath, depending upon the degree of orthodoxy or the rabbinical school followed.

RITUAL

For the Jew, to understand the glory and majesty of Yahweh with a pure and contemplative mind is an essential pursuit. To this end prayers are a key factor and are often said three times a day. Prayers are offered in the synagogue with the community or appointed prayer at home. Jewish prayers are prescribed although personal prayers may be offered. There are prayers for the home, for Sabbath worship, for children and for the dead. Jewish prayer embraces elements of petition, thanksgiving, praise, confession, sustaining and healing. Prayer which recognizes Yahweh's justice and mercy, emphasizes his willingness to listen and help and relieves the faithful of guilt over human sin. This is particularly relevant for the ill.

Stories of infertile women conceiving and of persons with terminal illness being healed after persistent prayer by the congregation help to encourage the patient. However, when in spite of such praying tragedy does occur, the prayers are still seen to be answered. To the Jew, God's will is the ultimate blessing and the prayers offered may not have been according to his will.

There are special festivals and days of fasting that have a bearing on the needs and behavior of a patient.

Judaism is the first of the great monotheistic religions of the world. Around 2000 BCE, Abraham, who was of Sumerian background, came out from Mesopotamia to settle in the Palestine area of the Levant. Between 1700 and 1200 BCE, the descendants of his grandson, Israel, were enslaved in Egypt. Moses miraculously led the children of Israel, escaping the slavery, into forty years of wilderness wanderings before settling down, according to the promise of God, in Palestine. During these years, by divine revelation Moses received the Jewish law—including the Ten Commandments—which has become the basis of the religion. Numerous other laws or traditions have been amassed as interpretations and applications of those laws. The basic law is the Torah, or the Pentateuch, which is found in the first five books of the Old Testament; a portion is read every Sabbath.

The Sabbath should be observed as a day of rest. Some strict Orthodox Jews will prefer not to write or switch on or off electric appliances on the Sabbath. If bed light, radio or television is turned on for them it is appreciated. The majority of Jews would accept normal hospital routine.

Pastoral and spiritual care

Visiting the sick is a supreme commandment for followers of the Jewish faith. It is incumbent not only on family members, but on all Jews, especially those who are friends or neighbors of the sick. It should be undertaken in a genuine spirit of warm and practical concern for the needs of the patients, giving them reassurance and comfort in the hours of pain and weakness. The best help often is prayer—for the sick and with the sick.

Rabbis gratefully appreciate the cooperation of hospital staff and Jewish colleagues in the ministry in assisting them by notifications, particularly of emergencies, and in other practical ways.

DIET

Dietary requirements of Jewish hospital patients will depend on the degree of observance customary in their homes. Those patients who uphold

the special dietary laws (*Kashrut*) will do so also
in hospital. Very briefly, these laws refer to the
provision of kosher food—special slaughtering
and preparation of meat, separation of milk and
meat foods, forbidden food, etc. In the period of
Passover, avoidance of all leaven and the provision of unleavened bread (*matzah*) are essential.

To obviate any difficulties for such observing
in hospitals, the following points are important:

- In cooperation with hospital staff, and with
  medical approval, the family concerned may
  be allowed to bring kosher food into the hospital.
- Milk and meat are usually not eaten at the
  same meal. Up to six hours may be required
  between eating meat and dairy products.
- Some patients may be satisfied with the provisions of vegetarian food, including dairy
  foods.
- A kosher meals service—if and when available—provides certain prepackaged meals by
  private arrangement (contact a rabbi or synagogue for information).
- In cases of danger to life, dietary laws are tem-
  porarily suspended.

- The assistance of a Jewish rabbi is particularly desirable and should be sought by dietitians at hospitals where patients have food problems.

CARE OF THE ILL AND DYING

A basic tenet of Judaism emphasizes that nothing must be allowed to stand in the way of preserving or prolonging life. Sabbath observance may be waived if necessary to assist a person whose life is in danger.

God himself is the supreme physician, "Who healeth the broken-hearted and bindeth up their wounds" (Psalm 147:3). Nevertheless, it is readily conceded that the divine healer does his work through mortals, and high respect is shown to members of the medical profession, following Ben Sira's famous utterance: "Honor a physician according to thy need of him, with the honors due unto him; for verily the Lord created him" (Ecclesiasticus 38:1–2).

Faith healing as it is understood in a specific sense by some Christians is foreign to and unknown within Judaism.

It is the doctor's duty to prolong life, so euthanasia is contrary to Jewish teachings. No *direct action to hasten death is permitted.* A patient on life support systems should remain on them until death. All active treatment should be maintained.

The Jewish religion does not recognize the concept of sacrament in the sense in which it is used by Christians. A person approaching death is encouraged to confess his or her sins before God (*Viddui*, or confession) and to evoke God's forgiveness. No confessor is needed, in the Jewish view, since only God can absolve sin. The shortest formula is "May my death atone for my transgressions," but this and other more elaborate wordings are best prompted and recited with the dying by a rabbi in attendance.

It is a basic tenet of Judaism that a dying person should not be left alone. When the end approaches, the last paragraph of the confession should be recited, especially the first line of the *shema*: "Hear O Israel, the Lord our God, the Lord is One."

The reading of Psalm 23 and the saying of the prayer (the entire *shema*) may be desired.

If at all possible, a minister of the Jewish faith (hospital chaplain or local rabbi or reverend) should be called in time to attend the needs of the dying patient.

Handling the deceased body—Death is presumed to occur when breathing appears to have stopped. When it is finally established, the eyes and mouth are gently closed (preferably by a near relative).

When life has departed, the arms and hands are extended at the side of the body. The lower jaw is bound up. The body is then placed on the floor with the feet toward the door and is covered with a sheet, while a lighted candle is placed close to the head.

The body must not be moved on the Sabbath (from Friday evening sunset to Saturday evening sunset, plus 30 minutes approximately). If death occurs in a hospital or nursing home, and no fellow Jews are available to carry out these services, the deceased may be carried out by hospital staff.

There is in most Jewish communities a special association, called *Chevra Kadisha* (Holy Brotherhood), which concerns itself with the burial of the dead. It is essential that this association, which functions as the Jewish burial society, be notified immediately when a death occurs.

The *Chevra* will take charge of all arrangements from the moment of notification. It will, in particular, remove the dead and will see to all other rites: ritual purification, including washing, shrouds, provision of the coffin, and all further funeral arrangements.

It will not operate on Sabbaths and festivals, but special provisions apply once the association is contacted.

Orthodox Jews are always buried in special Jewish burial grounds. Some liberal Jews may choose cremation.

AUTOPSIES, TRANSFUSIONS, TRANSPLANTS

It is forbidden in Jewish law to carry out an autopsy to ascertain the cause of death unless it is ordered by civil authorities. Dissection, including dissection for organs for donation is regarded as dishonoring the human body. Some Jewish authorities, however, do not object to organ transplants provided that no organ is removed until death has been established.

The chief Rabbinate of the State of Israel sanctions a postmortem examination when it is legally required, when in the opinion of three doctors the cause of death cannot otherwise be ascertained, when it might help or save the lives of others suffering from similar maladies* or in case of certain hereditary diseases. This ruling would be broadly applicable in all Jewish communities. Blood transfusions, if required and authorized by medical staff in the interests of the patient's welfare and life prolongation, are permitted. The patient's and family's preferences in these matters must be ascertained. Eye transplants are permitted by some authorities under certain safeguards on the grounds that they will help to restore sight to the living. An express request concerning this may be respected.

ABORTION AND FAMILY PLANNING

Contraception

Mechanical methods of contraception are not favored. Oral methods of birth control are acceptable. Sperm for IVF programs must be from the

---

*The Chief Rabbinate of Israel does not object to the use of bodies for anatomical dissection as required for medical studies, provided earlier voluntary consent has been given by the person concerned, and provided the dissected parts are carefully preserved for later burial.

husband. Orthodox Jews are more strict in their attitudes, therefore all forms of sterilization are forbidden. Reformed Jews are more accepting.

Abortion is a complex problem in the Jewish Law with no clear-cut answer. The following points are essential:

- Up to the moment of the first signs of labor, the fetus is an organic part of the mother. The artificial termination of pregnancy—while not an act of murder—is strongly condemned on moral grounds, unless it can be justified for medical reasons (serious deformity, imbecility and similar causes).
- The fetus must be destroyed if this is the only way in which the mother's life can be saved.
- Abortion for economic reasons or when the child is unwanted is not permitted.

Circumcision

On the birth of a male child, the parents' rabbi should be notified to arrange the ritual circumcision. Any doubt about the child's health will delay the circumcision. The rite is conducted by a trained and medically certified religious person, often the local rabbi. Should the mother and child still be in the hospital, a private room should be made available. A *minyan*, or quorum (usually ten), of Jewish males should be present.

MODESTY

An Orthodox Jewess will dress circumspectly and would prefer to have her body and limbs covered. She may refuse to permit herself to be uncovered for examination for teaching purposes. A woman may wear a wig or scarf so that others will not see her hair.

Male staff may attend female patients within the rules and framework of routine hospital arrangements that safeguard accepted standards of decency and modesty. While this is broadly the accepted position, it is possible that some Jewish patients may still object for religious reasons, and in such rare cases hospital staff will undoubtedly show understanding and cooperation.

FIVE

Hinduism

Hinduism is probably the oldest of the recognized living religions. It is difficult to date its origins, but to suggest that it has been more than 4,000 years since its establishment would not be an overestimation.

Hinduism embraces a galaxy of gods and goddesses. Ancient Scriptures such as the Vedas, the Upanishads, the Brahmanas, the Bhagavad Gita and other epics, such as the Mahabharata and the Ramayana, contain rich stories of these deities.

Basically Hindus believe in an ultimate great spirit, Brahman (Atma). He may be worshipped in many forms. Then comes the *trimurti* consisting of Brahma, the creator; Vishnu, the preserver; and Shib (Shiva), the destroyer and regenerator of life. After these comes a myriad of *avatars* and other deities.

Each major deity represents certain aspects of human living such as the elephant-headed Ganesh, the god of wealth. At the back of the till storekeepers often keep a shrine to Ganesh, with incense burning, Saraswati is the goddess of learning and is worshipped at the commencement of the school year in most public schools and even homes where there are school-age children.

Certain areas of India place a greater emphasis upon a particular god or goddess. For instance the goddess Durga, the victor over evil, is the main deity worshipped in eastern India, particularly Bengal.

Originally the Hindu caste system was an ideal way of ensuring a living and employment for all. The castes were the first form of trade union or work guilds. In India the system is now illegal although some customs die hard.

The doctrine of *karma* (the moral law of cause and effect) influences many a Hindu's attitude to life. Hindus see life events as being due to their *karma*. Many interpret this as fatalism. *Karma* is the working out in this present life of something that happened in a past life. Strongly believing in reincarnation, they hold that present status and behavior have a bearing on existence in the next reincarnated life.

Hinduism may be looked upon as a philosophy that covers the whole of life, including health. *Ayurvedic* medicine, practiced for millennia, is still practiced today. A Hindu may show some reticence to follow protocol in the hospital in case it counters *ayurvedic* practice, which covers a regimen of regular diet, sleep, defecation, hygiene, clothing, exercise and sexual practice.

Practitioners of *ayurvedic* medicine are recognized as being experts, who are honest and trustworthy. Such trust and confidence may be transferred from the *ayurvedic* doctor to the doctor of Western medicine.

Because of the belief in reincarnation, Orthodox Hindus are vegetarians. In reincarnation, the spirit of a newly deceased person may enter a dog, cow, chicken, even an egg. However, contact with Westernization sometimes weakens these beliefs and practices.

The Hindu's ultimate hope is to live such a good life in one of her or his many incarnations that she or he will eventually be absorbed into Brahman (Atma). By living a pure ethical life, loving and caring for fellow human beings and other creatures, "humans can realize God."

Hindu worship consists of a plethora of rituals that are focused in the family shrine, the local temple and a pilgrimage site. The household shrine is set up within the home or in the court-yard, or it may be the *tulsi* (basil) bush growing in the courtyard, around which the instruments for worship are arranged. At dusk each evening the women usually perform *puja* around the shrine, their distinctive wail resounding around the village accompanied by the ringing of bells and the waving of incense. Prayers are offered for the personal needs of the family. The local tem-ple is visited by some on a regular basis and on particular festival days for the temple deity when the whole community joins in. Places of special pilgrimage are found from Amarnath in the Kash-mir Himalayas to Kamakhya in Assam to Varanasi by the Ganges.

The times of *puja*, or worship, are important as worshippers believe they are encountering the forces that influence the physical and material world—the worshipper's world. Such worship practices are not possible in the hospital ward. The family, particularly the women, will visit their own temple or conduct *puja* around the family altar at home.

NAMES

Hindu patients are likely to have three or four names, according to their background. In the north it is usual to have a given or personal (not Christian) name followed by a second one, possibly the father's given name or the name of a deity or a title, e.g., Bipendra (father's name), Chandra (moon), Krishna (god) or Kumar (prince). The third name is the family name, which usually indicates the caste, e.g., Chakraborty (brahman or priestly caste), Agawalla (merchant caste). In south India four names may be used: great-grandfather, grandfather, father and given name. The last name should always be used for medical records.

DIET AND FASTING

For most Hindus diet is important. Most will not eat beef; vegetarian Hindus eat no white or red meats, no eggs, and nothing that is produced from animals. Some, however, may eat cottage cheese, yogurt, even eggs, and drink milk. Tomato or similar sandwiches are safe to offer a Hindu patient. There are certain other eating taboos with certain types of illnesses.

🖎 *Always inquire carefully of a Hindu's dietary needs.*

Fasting is not considered obligatory in the hospital during festival periods. There are those few who may insist on fasting, but even in this case tea, hot milk, salt-free salads and fruits are permitted. At the end of the festival relatives may bring in food and sweetmeats that have been offerings for the *puja*.

RITUALS

Birth

Birth practices vary. In the higher caste families the mother is forced to rest for forty days after the birth.

For the pious Hindu three ceremonies take place before birth:

- to promote conceptions;
- to procure a male child;
- to ensure the safety of the child in the womb.

In the home birth, a ceremony involving *mantras* (prayer) said in the baby's ear, putting a mixture of honey and *ghee* (clarified butter) on the baby's tongue, and naming her or him is followed. The name is kept secret until later.

This birth scenario is not possible in a hospital. However, the mantra and name may be whispered in the baby's ear as soon as possible after birth by the mother or father. It requires only one or two minutes.

Where hospital procedures insist on moving the baby into a nursery it may require considerable persuasion to pacify the separated mother.

Ritual ablutions and washing

Physical cleansing is associated with spiritual cleansing, hence its importance to the Hindu. As with most people of Asian origin, there will be the need for water for washing after use of the toilet. A container of water should be available in the toilet and when a bedpan is used. Hindus, like Muslims, prefer showers or running water to baths.

AUTOPSIES, TRANSFUSIONS, TRANSPLANTS

There are no religious objections to such procedures. Autopsies generally are acceptable although Hindus are happier if they can be avoided. Only normal consent procedures for organ donation or transplants need to be followed.

However, some may object strongly to post-mortems and organ donations, desiring the body to remain intact.

ABORTION AND FAMILY PLANNING

Hinduism places no restrictions on the use of contraception. The importance of a male child to a family may put pressure upon the woman to continue with additional pregnancies until a son is born. If there are medical or financial reasons for the limitation of the size of the family, then the husband should be involved in any such information sharing and decision making.

The fetus is considered a living entity; applying logic to the belief in *Ahisma* (nonviolence), it seems that abortion would be abhorred. However, abortions are accepted for several reasons—particularly female fetuses. In this technological age, tests to determine sex of the fetus are performed. Frequently the female fetus is aborted because males are preferred and daughters are considered financial burdens, particularly when it comes to marriage.

CARE OF THE ILL AND DYING

In an area with a strong Hindu community, a Hindu priest is able to help in matters of worship (*puja*). Accepting death philosophically is a trait of Hinduism; the priest, if available, fulfills the role of facilitating such acceptance. A devout Hindu may desire to read the Hindu Scriptures, particularly the Bhagavad Gita.

Other rituals that may be performed are the tying of thread around the neck or wrist of the dying patient, the sprinkling of Ganges water over the patient, the placing of a leaf from the sacred basil (*tulsi*) bush on the tongue, or the bringing of money for the patient to touch before it is offered as alms to the needy.

Some patients may want to lie on the floor to be closer to the earth with incense burning around them. Patience is required in handling them. Others may want to die at home. Every reasonable consideration should be given to such a request.

Handling of the deceased body

Following death, the family should be consulted before the body is handled as the family may wish to wash and dress the deceased. Where such consultation is not possible, disposable gloves should be used to close the eyes and straighten the limbs and remove jewelry.

Sacred threads* and other religious objects should not be removed. The body—unwashed, as this is part of the family funeral rites—should be wrapped in a plain sheet or shroud. It will be cremated.

Hindu practice varies widely. The above is only a general outline of what may be expected. Always ask the patient or eldest son or other senior male relatives what the patient's wishes are or would be.

MODESTY

Hindu women may indicate a preference to be treated or examined by a female doctor.

Efforts should be made to avoid the embarrassment to a patient being sent for tests in a short hospital gown.

---

*The sacred thread is presented to a son of the brahman (priestly) caste. It is a white thread tied around the waist and up over the shoulder. The patient should be cremated wearing the sacred thread.

→ SIX ←

Jainism

The principle guru of Jainism (died ca. 526 BCE)
was a prince of the Kshatriya caste of Hinduism
similar to his contemporary Siddhartha Gautama,
the founder of Buddhism. He is best known by
the name Mahavira (the Great Hero). There is no
claim that he founded Jainism. Rather he was the
twenty-fourth *Tirthankara* (Fordmaker).

This eternal universe has cycles of advances
and developments followed by regression and
degradation on all fronts. During those times of
negative reversal a *Tirthankara* appears to
amend the situation. This cycle of decline lasts
about 21,000 years. For this purpose, these
Tirthankaras arise to reclaim humanity from the
downward spiral by founding a new religion appropriate to the period. There were twenty-three

Tirthankaras before Mahavira. Jainism will gradually disappear as the next evil cycle begins to destroy the moral fabric of that society.

Jainism embraced the philosophy of early Hinduism that saw two states of reality:

1. *Purusha*—the changeless, eternal, wise, pure and true liberated free self. *Purusha* was described by some as the representative of the ideal human.
2. *Prakriti* (matter)—the impermanent appearance of reality in time.

The human aspects of *Prakriti* include: self-consciousness, intelligence, sense perception, etc. The material manifestations of *Prakriti* are seen in fire, water, earth, etc.

Living in this world of matter, humans are living in a state of *samsara*; i.e., "the ocean of suffering." The Jains strive for liberation from this *samsara* by avoiding reincarnation (rebirth). This is done by self-effort along the road to discovering the *Purusha* within one's self. It may require many rebirths to achieve this pure ethical life. Rebirths may continue for up to 700,000 years. This fits in with the belief in cause and effect, or *karma*: As you sow, so you reap.

Jiva, or soul, is a living substance integral to all life forms, including humans and the plant and animal worlds. *Jiva* provides hope for the Jains because it is through the *jiva* that the ideal eternal nature is able to overcome the miseries of the earthly life. The Jains see *karma* as a material substance that flows into the *jiva* on account of actions or deeds. *Karma* is the soul in bondage. Bad *karma* from a previous and present life may be eliminated by self-mortification, fasting and the following of the "Three Jewels": right action, right faith and right knowledge. These are implemented by: meditation, regular fasting, confession and repentance of sin to a guru. If Jain gurus are contactable they should be called to allow for such confession to be heard, if desired by the patient.

Jains believe that the only means of escape from the ties of this material world and release from the *karmic* cycle is by self-discipline and nonviolence. Only humans with positive *karma* are able to reach *nirvana* (the eternal state of blessedness). When this happens, *jiva* is freed from individuality and desires, and is released from the effects of *karma*.

Thus a Jain endeavors to live according to three ethical principles:

1. *Nonviolence, or Ahisma.* This means the nonharming of any living organism. Humans are on the same level of existence and status as all living creatures. Reverence for all life is essential to the faith of a Jain. A Jain monk may be seen sweeping the path in front of him as he walks to avoid the killing of an insect. Even the smallest microbes are considered to be on a similar path to gain *Purusha* status. To kill or harm anything builds up bad *karma*. In regard to interpersonal relations, any negative thought or action against another can emotionally hurt or physically harm the other. Jains avoid pursuits such as farming as it inevitably results in the killing of insects, bacteria and even weeds and other plants in the soil. Ploughing hurts the oxen or buffaloes used, their necks become calloused from the yoke and they are beaten into action. Hence Jains are found in occupations such as bureaucrats, merchants, office workers, monks and nuns. Some Jains may wear face masks to prevent the inhalation by nose or mouth of airborne microbes. Jains, in many cities of India have established elaborate cow shelters for aged or stray cattle. They are housed and fed in brick and tile compounds with great care. This is to prevent them being mistreated or harmed in any way.

2. *Non-attachment, or aparigraha.* Attachment to and accumulation of possessions promotes avarice, covetousness and selfishness. For this reason, the first twenty-three *Tirthankaras* are depicted in paintings or statutes without clothes. Some monks go around in public naked. Monks and nuns must obtain their necessities for life by depending upon the faithful to supply. They will not buy or cook food. All meals are provided by others. It is believed that by nonattachment more of the essentials of life will be available for the poor, the needy, the disabled and underprivileged of the world.

3. *Relativity, or anekantwad.* Jains are generally open-minded, nondogmatic and accepting people who believe that any issue or event can be interpreted differently from different aspects. All things are relative to the perspective from which they are being viewed or experienced. Jains may see love for a personal God as an irrelevant attachment likely to produce bad *karma.* Thus Jains worship their *Tirthankaras* who are not considered to be gods. Such worship is considered merely as veneration without supplication or seeking blessing from them in any form. Such veneration is aimed at inspiring the desire to emulate the pure life of the *Tirthankara* being hon-

ored. Thus worship is relative to the intention.
The breaking of the cycle of reincarnations is only
possible through self effort and not by favor of a
Tirthankara.

DIET

Jains are very strict vegetarians so the consumption of meat or animal products in any form is
considered to be the killing of a creature. Thus all
forms of flesh are taboo for Jains. Biscuits, cakes
and other food made using eggs are also forbidden. Eggs are considered to contain a living organism. A Jain may request that water for consumption be filtered or strained to keep it free
from microorganisms.

ORGAN DONATIONS, TRANSFUSIONS, TRANSPLANTS

Generally these are unacceptable because the
procedures would involve pain and harm to the
body of the donor or the organs of the recipient.

CARE OF THE ILL AND DYING

The Jain must burn up as much bad *karma* as
possible. This may be done by strict self-disci-

pline including patiently bearing pain and suffering. For this reason only, minimum or no medication may be requested. The patient may see medication as a means of stopping the flow of good *karma*.

Austerity and asceticism can affect rebirth by this burning away of bad *karma*. So at death, a Jain must be in full control of the body. Fasting cleans out the body, so that the mind is able to concentrate on the spiritual destiny in the next life. The ideal way to die is in meditation. Because a Jain may desire to fast and be left to meditate when facing serious illness and impending death, she or he will express the desire to be free from all painkilling and sedative medication. Some Jains on being informed or becoming aware of approaching death may take a vow of total abstinence from food (*santharo*) and die of voluntary starvation (*sallekhana*). Being aware of this will save the patient from severe distress if staff attempt to force-feed the patient. The staff should try to make the patient as comfortable as possible without sedation to facilitate concentration on meditation.

Conditions are different for Jains in a Western setting. Therefore it is essential that attending staff should ascertain beforehand the wishes of

the patient and the family as to their desires as
death approaches.

POSTDEATH PROCEDURES

The family will arrange the removal of the body.
In India, the dead are neither interred nor have a
normal cremation. The body is taken to a tower,
known as "The Tower of Silence." At the top of
this tower, the body is placed on a grate. Scav-
enging vultures come and pick the flesh off the
bones, which then fall below through the grate
into a furnace where they are cremated.

SEVEN

Sikhism

In Hinduism, the power of ritual, the effectiveness of *mantras,* and the sacrificial system unify the people under the power of the priests. Mahavira, the founder of Jainism, and Siddhartha Gautama, founder of Buddhism, argued that the priestly dominance did not permit the ordinary worshippers to understand truth and receive enlightenment or liberation. Hence Jainism and Buddhism separated from Hinduism a few centuries before the Christian era.

Two thousand years later Guru Nanak (1469–1539) saw the caste system as dangerous and other elements as too complicated, and also perceived that ritual dominated. Influenced by Islam (and perhaps Christianity), he recognized the confusion created by a multiplicity of gods. His reform renounced the priesthood and the caste system, and established monotheism. He also gave women a new status. Equality of all people became a focal point. Sikhism is more than a reform of Hinduism; Nanak and his nine successors developed an independent religion. They retained the Hindu concept that reincarnation lasts until true understanding and unity with the divine is accomplished.

The writings of ten prophets or gurus form the Sikh Scriptures known as Guru Grant Sahab, or Ad Granth. Sikhs use this as their teacher as there is no priesthood. The Sikh *Gurdwara* (temple) is managed by the community, who oversee all religious and social services.

Guru Gobind Singh (1666–1708) was the last of the gurus. It was he who developed the militaristic character of the Sikhs. He also built on Nanak's emphasis upon the equality of the sexes, which differed greatly from Hinduism and Islam.

Gobind Singh takes the credit for establishing the wearing of the five *K* symbols by every initiated Sikh male or female. There should be an awareness of these symbols when nursing or treating a Sikh, to avoid embarrassment or mis-understanding. They are:

Kesh—uncut hair. Usually it is left long and tied into a bun. The men cover it with a turban; elderly pious Sikh women may wear black turbans.

Kangha—a comb. A small semicircular comb to keep the bun in place. Even if for some medical or surgical reason it cannot be kept in the bun it should always remain close to the patient's body.

Kara—a steel bangle. Originally used to protect the wrist from cuts from the bowstring, it now symbolizes the unity of God. During surgery it, as with a wedding ring, should not be removed but covered. Where the arm on which it is worn is involved in the procedure, the bangle can be put on the other wrist, worn pinned to the pajamas or put under the pillow.

Kirpan—a short dagger. It symbolizes the readiness of the Sikh to fight against injustice and to protect the oppressed. Some Sikhs still carry a real dagger. More commonly worn as a brooch or pendant, *Kirpan* may also be engraved on the *Kangha*. Sikhs who wear the

Kirpan will wear it all the time in bed, in the shower and in the hospital. To remove it will cause great distress to the patient. If in exceptional circumstances it cannot be worn against the body, it must be kept in sight. The reasons must be carefully *explained to the patient and relatives and be understood* by them.

Kaccha—white underpants or shorts. Originally these were knee-length for ease of movement in battle. They also symbolize modesty and sexual morality. At childbirth a woman may insist on having one leg in a *Kaccha*. In changing *Kacchas* one leg must remain in the old or soiled *Kaccha* until the other leg is in the clean one. This should be observed when giving a bed bath or a bedpan.

NAMES

The Sikhs usually have three names. There is the given name first, e.g., Mahinda for a male or Amrit for a female. Then comes a title, Singh for all men and Kaur for all women. A family name such as Gill or Bhuller then follows.

Thus a man's name may be Mahinda Singh Gill. He will often register as Mahinda Gill Singh;

similarly a woman as Amrit Bhuller Kaur. To keep medical records from confusion, it is wiser to register patients under the family name as Gill, M. S. or Bhuller, A. K. A husband is usually known as Mr. Singh and his wife as Mrs. Kaur—never Mrs. Singh.

RITUAL

For devout Sikhs prayer is important. Normally a Sikh will rise early, bathe and say prayers before breakfast. In the hospital, privacy is essential when saying prayers. The following should be made available if possible, even for a dying patient:

- the opportunity for an early shower or
- quick bed sponge before prayers at breakfast;
- the pulling of curtains to ensure privacy while praying.

DIET AND FASTING

There is a wide range of practices. Most of the official Sikh stances relating to food and drink are now observed, but with varying degrees of strictness.

Some common restrictions ban:

- alcohol
- *halal* meat, i.e., Muslim-slaughtered meats
- eggs, for many women who are vegetarian
- beef or pork
- tobacco smoking

Since not all Sikhs observe the above restrictions, each Sikh patient should be asked about special requirements.

A few Sikhs may wish to fast when there is a full moon.

Ritual ablutions and washing

Running water for washing and showering with the provision of water near the toilet or with the bedpan are requirements.

Water is also required for washing the hands and mouth before eating.

Birth

Sikhs consider a woman to not be at her best after childbirth and she must be protected. It is believed that she is susceptible to chills and back pain at such time. She will not wish to bathe for a few days to avoid these risks. Normally a nursing mother is allowed forty days rest after the birth. Hospital routine may seem to run counter to this.

Separation of mothers from the baby into a nursery may meet with resistance. Tactful explanations will be necessary if this is hospital procedure.

Relatives and friends will want to see the baby as soon after the birth as possible and gifts of clothing are usually tried on the baby. Gentle persuasion to just leave the gift will be needed by the staff, or restraint may be necessary.

ABORTION AND FAMILY PLANNING

Abortions are acceptable only if the mother's life is at risk.

There are generally no objections to contraception and family planning.

AUTOPSIES, TRANSFUSIONS, TRANSPLANTS

There are no religious objections to any of these.

Careful and neat suturing of the body postautopsy is required in case the family insists on washing the body prior to cremation. Careless presentation of the body is likely to cause great distress.

CARE OF THE ILL AND DYING

Sikhs may derive comfort from hearing passages of Guru Grant Sahab when dying. If patients are unable to read, a relative or any practicing Sikh may do it.

Because of their belief in reincarnation, Sikhs are not fearful of death. They believe they can alter the cycle by living a good life and accumulating rewards or punishments in the next life.

Handling of the deceased body

Non-Sikhs may attend the body at death. It is essential to see that the five *K*s or symbols are in place and have not been mistreated.

No hair should be cut or trimmed. A nurse may close the eyes and straighten out the limbs and wrap the body in a plain sheet or shroud.

Cremation takes place as soon as possible (except when there is a stillborn child, then the child may be buried). Some women will not eat until after the cremation. Women wear white as a sign of mourning. After ten days another ceremony, called the *Bhog*, is held to formally end the mourning period.

MODESTY

Most women would prefer to be examined by a female doctor, but they will not object to a male doctor's examination if a female nurse is present.

The removal of the *Kaccha* (undershorts) from either male or female may cause great embarrassment as will the removal of the turban.

EIGHT

Buddhism

A royal prince, named Siddhartha, was born in the sixth century BCE in what is now the Himalayan kingdom of Nepal. This prince observed that most people experienced suffering of one kind or another and understood that people sought unsuccessfully for happiness. He left the comfort of palace and home to seek the truth that would bring true happiness.

After several years of futile search, a sudden inspiration took hold of him while he was sitting, meditating under a banyan tree at Gaya in North India. The truth burned within him that happiness came from changing the self from the inside. This became known as "Enlightenment." He then was given the title of Buddha, which means "the enlightened one."

His expansive teaching life followed. He taught that greed, hatred and delusion destroyed happiness. Wisdom and compassion were the secrets to happiness. The ultimate state, *nirvana*, which is in some ways similar to what Christians call heaven, can be attained only through an absence of desire and the achievement of perfection, and no awareness of separate identity.

His eightfold path to enlightenment was: right view or understanding, right thought, right speech, right action, right livelihood, right effort, right mindfulness, right meditation. Buddhists believe in reincarnation until the absence of desire is attained. They do not believe in a god as creator, and worship is the acknowledgment of an ideal.

Buddhism in contrast to Hinduism claims that liberation from *karma* can also be achieved not entirely by self-realization but by smothering all desires that lead to a continuing in the state of *samara*. *Samsara* is the cycle of suffering experienced through being reborn on earth according to the *karma* built up in the previous life. Meditation is able to assist in eradicating desire. When desire has been eliminated entirely *nirvana* is reached. Meditation—in particular, meditation on death—becomes important on the road to *nir-vana*. This is never more important than when facing a medical crisis.

Death is accepted as a natural step into a further life by being reborn into another body unless the Buddha nature has been fully experienced. Pain and suffering is accepted as part of this process. This death preparation process, according to Mahayana Buddhism, includes eight stages and may not be completed until a day or two after breathing ceases. The minimum movement of the body after the declaration of clinical death should be recognized by the staff for this reason.

Relatives desire to be informed of the immanence of death so that they can make the necessary preparations. If possible, they prefer the patient to die at home. The possibility of such an arrangement should be pursued by health-care providers.

In the health-care facility, relatives may desire to maintain a constant vigil for the peace and comfort of the patient. Other patients may prefer solitude in order to meditate. The patient's desire should always be ascertained and should not be dictated by the relatives. Remember, anticipation of rebirth is the important focus when facing death. Health-care staff's awareness of this should be given high priority in their care of the patient at this time.

Buddhism still embraces much of the worship, teaching and beliefs of Hinduism. The philosophy of Buddhism—of prayers, purifications, meditation, retreats and virtuous living—has attracted many people from the Western world.

DIET AND FASTING

As Buddhists are found in countries with a wide range of climates, diets vary. Many Buddhists are vegetarians because the eating of meat entails suffering to the slain animal. Some may even consider, as some Hindus do, that an animal contains a reincarnated human spirit. An awareness of the possible need for a vegetarian diet is important for those Buddhist patients.

Festivals and days of fasting vary among the schools of Buddhism. On the special festival days the patient may request to eat before noon and not after.

RITUALS

Birth

Apart from babies born into aristocratic families, no special ceremonies are performed after the birth of a child. No special rituals are required in trauma-related cases.

Ritual ablutions and washing

Buddhist Scriptures have no special instructions concerning washing and cleansing after attending to toilet functions. Buddhists come from various countries with varying customs, so their requirements may vary. Patients should be asked if they have special needs.

AUTOPSIES, TRANSFUSIONS, TRANSPLANTS

Buddhists have no objections to autopsies, blood transfusions or transplants. These would be considered as being of assistance in the relief of suffering or the acquiring of knowledge that may help others. The only condition is that life is not destroyed in the pursuit of these. Active euthanasia is therefore forbidden.

ABORTION

For the same reason abortion is generally condemned.

Similarly, family planning may be considered as interfering with one's destiny; its practice is therefore conditional upon the couple's background.

CARE OF THE ILL AND DYING

The health-care staff may be either male or female except where the patient is a monk or nun (sister). In such cases, staff of the same sex should be considered for the care of the patient.

Buddhists appreciate a visit from a monk or sister if they are available. Ask the patient for the contact person.

Buddhists often spend time in meditation before a shrine. In the hospital the shrine may simply be an image of Buddha. Staff should be aware that the patient is in meditation when a picture of the Buddha is in view of the patient. Space for such meditation should be allowed as it is a factor in physical well-being and recuperation. There are two conflicting emphases of Buddhism that affect the patient: the relief of pain and suffering and the importance of "mindfulness," that is, being mentally alert and aware.

As far as possible, there is a need for a Buddhist to have a clear mind during their preparation for death. Therefore, they may refuse any painkilling or sedative medication. The patient must be kept informed of the effects of any medications that have been prescribed so as not to generate anxiety should they begin to lose their ability to concentrate while meditating. Their right to refuse medication should be accepted.

For the Buddhist, earthly life is a path of spiritual progression and provides opportunities to purify the self of any sin or wrong thought in pursuit of attaining the Buddha nature as achieved by Gautama. To hasten death by any means including euthanasia is to destroy further opportunities for further spiritual achievements.

Handling of the deceased body

No formal or ritualistic functions are prescribed for the body. If a monk is present, he may (depending upon the school of Buddhism) recite prayers for about one hour. The prayers do not have to be recited in the presence of the body. Therefore it is helpful for the relatives if a monk is informed as soon as possible after the death.

The monk should be of the same school or tradition and background if possible.

Some Buddhist cultures may insist on the completion of a prayer ritual before the body is moved. Others will have the relatives touch the crown of the head before any transfer of the body as the crown is said to be the place from which the conscious is said to leave the body. Once the consciousness has left the body there is no objection to any autopsy or use of the body for scientific purposes. Chinese Buddhists may object to this.

Normal hospital procedure in preparation of the body after death is acceptable.

A Buddhist prefers cremation and that final disposal takes place between three and seven days after death.

Where Buddhist rites cannot be observed, any person may conduct the final service. There should be no reference to God, prayers, or doctrines of other religions. A memorial eulogy is accepted practice and a few passages from a Buddhist Scripture may be read, if possible. If a Christian minister or priest is requested to conduct such a service, this should be considered seriously. She or he should be well prepared if the invitation is accepted.

NINE

China's Complementary Religions

Taoism, Buddhism, and Confucianism in China, and Jainism and Buddhism in India, all had their origins around five hundred years before Christianity.

In the Far Eastern countries of Japan, China and Korea, religion, like all other major developments, sprang from its primal roots. The common thread of indigenous religion seen in these countries was ancestor worship. Ancestors were revered and worshipped, with the living still feeling strong bonds with those who went before them. This homage to ancestors after the funeral and mourning rites took the form of sacrifices. These rituals are called *li* in the belief that having been given proper honor, ancestors will help and inspire their descendants to live more noble lives and to deal with personal problems. Nature deities and other deities were also worshipped at shrines and temples. In the earlier days, shamanism was the foundational root from which Chinese society developed later religious beliefs. The shaman was the mediator between the spirits and the people.

Archeologists have traced religious origins back to the Shang Dynasty (ca. 1523–1027 BCE). From an early date the Chinese believed that each person has a spiritual component. At death, efforts were made to keep the spirit within the body by plugging up all the orifices. This developed into prayers that the spirits of the deceased ancestors intercede on their behalf to the supernatural beings that ruled the universe. Thus ancestor worship was established. In time, regular sacrifices were made to these ancestor spirits.

This led to the belief that humans possessed *hun*, the conscious personality of a living human, and *po*, the spirit animating the body. This *po* spirit remains with the body after death. The *hun* continues to actively utilize all the powers of the conscious intellect and will in the heavenly courts of the Emperor of Heaven. The funeral ritual is a rite to summon back the *hun* spirit so that the deceased relative becomes a celestial being with *po* descending to the nether world in what might be called "soul sleep." The celestial *hun* is then able to be offered sacrifices by the survivors in order to gain help in living a life of virtue.

Confucianism is considered more a philosophy rather than a religion.

Five hundred years after the Shang Dynasty, Confucianism and Taoism began to capture the Chinese mind. Each increased its influence over the Chinese population.

TAOISM

Unlike many other religions Taoism cannot point to one person or supernatural event as its inspirational foundation. It has developed an evolutionary philosophical process over a long period by many teachers who were not adverse to assimilate, adapt or reform from outside practices. A Taoist is a follower of "the Way"—*Tao* means "the Way." Early Taoists recognized two opposing forces in the world. They saw them as negative and positive poles, which they called *yin* and *yang*. When they are reconciled they provide the "Way" to Heaven. *Yin* also represents the female, receptive and dark aspects. *Yang* is the male, assertive and light pole. These contending forces are responsible for the continuous changes that are experienced by all life. For man to oppose these changes is to act contrary to the natural way of the universe. Man-made changes are artificial. Taoism has adopted the principle of moving with the flow of change by the practice of *wu wei* or nonaction, avoiding action contrary to nature. Taoism adapts to, rather than strives against, the environment.

This philosophy of following the way of least resistance to these *yin* and *yang* forces is likened to water meandering down the natural contours of the landscape to the ocean— hence the appellation "the Water-course Way."

This need to balance the *yin* and *yang* is applied to man's need to have a balance between body, mind and spirit. By balancing all the components of a person's life it enables the achievement of harmony and the avoidance of disharmony. It is a balance of spiritual perception and material action.

Flowing through nature is the energy or *chi*. *Chi* oscillates between the poles of *yin* and *yang*. The right control of *chi* is important on the way to achieving immortality, which is the ultimate goal of the Taoist. The Taoist employs all the powers or energy of body, mind and spirit to achieve *Tao*. This involves the art of stilling the mind, emptying itself of the desires and longings of the material world. By this, the follower of *Tao* accepts death and illness as an integral part of existence as birth, growth and gain. Loss and gain are all essential to attain tranquility of spirit through this *yin* and *yang*.

To maintain this balance or harmony of body, mind and spirit, Chuang-tzu accepts the need to practice physical exercise, secure internal change and receive spiritual revelation. Meditation, the fine arts and martial arts are methods used to achieve these ends. The intent of these is to improve mental and general health, physical agility, the discipline of moving meditation and the flow of *chi* through the body.

The *Tao* has been described as the egg, root, womb and mother of life. The person whose life is surrendered to the selfless, natural rhythm of life is renewed in death by returning to *Tao*, its origin of life.

Tai Chi is the use of rhythmic exercise as a form of internal martial art to calm the body. Meditation provides the medium for stilling and emptying the mind to affect change so that the spirit is able to listen to the revelatory silence or enable the perfect stillness of the mental void.

When all this is harmonized and death envelops the body the consciousness reaches immortality with the limitless void of the *Tao*.

The West appreciates Taoism from the above philosophical aspect. In the early centuries of the common era, Taoism also developed into a religious faith. Some began to believe that immortality could be attained through alchemy. In 150 CE, a shrine was built and dedicated to Lao-tzu who was one of the leaders in the pursuit of longevity in the health and exercise schools of Taoism. He became recognized as a celestial figure just as ancestors were venerated to ensure their guidance and daily assistance.

Taoism soon developed a system with revered deities, shrines, religious leaders, religious rites and fasting. It became the unchallenged state religion of China. It has never lost sight of the aim of maintaining a healthy mind and body by exercising a control that leads to longevity and immortality. To this end control was exercised by following a moral code of conduct. This included personal and social responsibility as well as sexual morality. Its message continued to stress compassion and harmony with nature. Ultimately a Taoist pantheon evolved into two streams—the Earlier Heaven Deities and the Later Heaven

Deities with Lao-tzu as the greatest. A rich mythology was also consolidated.

Several different schools of Taoism have arisen. Suffice to say their goal remains to attain immortality, which means a denial of the ego and the death of self. Immortality is the realization that we are part of the eternal "one" and that we embrace immortality beyond human life—the eternal state of transcendence.

MEDICAL IMPLICATIONS

The Taoist belief in *yin* and *yang* sees life holistically. Illness is an imbalance of *yin* and *yang*, or of a person's body, mind and spirit. Because of this, Taoists see sedatives and pain control measures as violations of the personal right to control or avoid the discipline or lessons that the gods want the patient to exercise or learn. Some medications may be refused; some may wish to combine folk medicine with Western medical treatment.

Because *yin* and *yang* are also associated with masculinity and femininity, as well as light and darkness, and depending on regional cultural background, Taoists may object to a homosexual member of the health team attending to them.

Such a person may be seen as bringing a conflicting imbalance into their hospitalization and countering the healing process.

DIET AND FOOD

The Taoist is normally a vegetarian but may eat meat if it is necessary for a balanced diet. Generally, Taoists will accept the hospital dietician's recommendations to maintain such a balance. While fasting is recognized by some followers of *Tao*, it is not regularly practiced. However as the patient is on the last stage of the journey to *Tao* they may see a need to restrict the expenditure of *chi* in the energy lost by the digestive system. The patient may indicate that they desire to fast or have only the minimum of food nourishment. The devout Taoist will want to conserve the maximum *chi* for the postdeath stage of the journey to *Tao*.

CARE OF THE ILL AND DYING

When the patient is diagnosed with a terminal or other serious medical condition, such information should be conveyed to the patient by a close relative and not directly by medical staff. As Chinese have strong familial ties it is considered appropriate that this procedure is followed. Medical staff must be aware of this. Even if a suspecting patient asks a nurse or doctor directly, they should not reveal the nature of the illness unless the relatives have been told and the relatives have conveyed it to the patient. Ancestor worship is ingrained deeply into Chinese culture; this reverence for elders requires as many relatives as possible to visit the patient not only to offer comfort and solace but to also receive blessings from the patient.

In the days prior to death, the patients will want to build up internal *chi* in readiness for a successful completion of their earthly journey. Health-care providers should be aware of this and provide as much time alone as possible for the patient to concentrate and meditate upon reaching *Tao*. This requires as comfortable a position as possible to meditate.

As the patient is dying

The whole of life is a spiritual journey to *Tao*. Death is part of that journey. *Yin* represents the earth pole; a Taoist may ask for assistance to be closer to the *yin* by being placed on a mat on the floor. Any rituals are usually performed by a son.

At the approach of death the relatives may remove their jewelry—a representation of material wealth—and form a circle around the patient's bed. Here *yin* and *yang* are present in the form of both male and female visitors. The men stand on the east as representing the *yang* and to the west the women—the *yin*. This is considered an additional vehicle to make the path easier for the patient.

AUTOPSIES, ORGAN DONATIONS, TRANSFUSIONS

Taoism provides no resistance to organ donations or blood transfusions. Autopsies will not be considered, particularly if it is for further knowledge about the patient's condition, the disease or purely for scientific purposes. As in most similar situations with other religions, cultural influences dictate. Therefore relatives' or the patient's wishes should be obtained prior to the demise if possible.

ABORTION

An abortion may be seen as human interference to terminate the earthly journey to *Tao* of the body, mind and spirit of the embryo. Abortion is not considered an option except if the life of the mother is endangered by the continuation of the pregnancy.

CARE OF THE ILL AND DYING

Handling the body

Upon death, the body is washed with a white washer by a relative and the body is placed with the head facing south. When the hair is combed, the comb is broken and collected with the other washing materials to be buried. Should a son or other family member not be present, a nurse may close the eyelids and wash the body.

The spirit and body

Differing views on the relation between the deceased spirit and the body prevail according to cultural background. Some believe that the spirit leaves the body to hover around the deceased until the burial; others say that the spirit stays with the body and is buried with it. The hospital staff should be very careful how they handle the body with relatives around regardless of the family's belief.

Funeral rites

The burial of the body takes place about seven days after the death, when a funeral service is conducted. However, one or more memorial services may be conducted before and after the funeral. Rituals take the form of prayers and incense burning; in China, paper offerings made in the form of houses, cars, etc., representing material possessions are burned during the funeral ceremony. In Western countries, these paper offerings may be substituted by flowers.

A period of one month is generally allowed for grieving by the relatives. During this time, dress and activities are expected to be in tune with the solemnity of the period. If any of the medical staff have had a good relationship with the patient or family, a visit to the home is very much appreciated.

CONFUCIANISM

Confucius (family name: Kung Fu-tzu) lived 551–479 BCE. His teaching was called "Teaching of the Scholars." He promoted a philosophy aimed at bringing harmony into human existence—it included ritual and applied ethics. Confucius, like the Taoists, was interested in promoting harmony within the individual. He also acknowledged that the opposing poles of *yin* and *yang* had to be kept in balance. They functioned together in human life and separated at death.

Confucianism is considered more a philosophy rather than a religion.

Confucius's principle concern was a balance in this life rather than considering deeply the life beyond death. Like Taoism, Confucianism acknowledges a unity between body, mind and spirit, daily life and ideal concepts. The transcendental and earthly although different interpenetrate. Taoism focuses upon the otherworldly—*Tao*; Confucianism centers on human life and the present. Hence the two religions may be said to complement each other.

Confucius considered human relationships were the key to harmony. Therefore, his emphasis was upon right, moral and ethical behavior to promote harmonious relations between individuals and within the community. Similar to Taoism, *li* was the virtue that practiced rites and duties honoring ancestors and deities. In these ceremonies to the gods and spirits, they are believed to be present observing all. Rites were not empty practices but were used to promote *jen* or self-improvement through right and ethical living toward all. Confucius cautioned against the overuse of rites, as they were to be taken as serious attempts to preserve harmony between humans, heaven and earth. Thus *li* goes beyond the mere practice of rituals.

The human spirit gives substance to human behavior. Within humans there is an inherent sense of good and evil. *Li* is intended to promote the good within the human spirit to balance the thoughts of the mind and the actions of the body that will result in ethical living. Confucius put what became the Christian's golden rule in the negative form. "Do not do to others what you would not do to yourself." This was meant to bring harmony into all human relationships— family, community and state. To live a good, clean ethical life is the basis of Confucian teaching.

The five cardinal virtues of Confucianism are: kindness, moral integrity, decorum, wisdom and sincerity. Therefore the characteristics of a Confucian should be: moderation, courtesy and self-control. A noble honorable character is superior to culture and wealth.

From the second century BCE to the second century CE Confucian teaching was accepted by the state.

Confucius and death

Death was not a concern of Confucius. As already indicated, Confucianism deals with the here and now. He discouraged any thought about the future life and gods. He is reported to have said, "If we are not yet able to serve man, how can we serve spiritual beings?" Man's focus must be making this world a better place through developing harmonious relations between all.

His support of ancestor worship came from his firm belief that this practice helped to maintain good relationships between the living and those that had gone ahead. Reverence for ancestors was a model for the way we should respect our contemporaries. Confucius's disciples emphasized this when they taught that the living should be treated with the same respect and service demonstrated in ancestor rituals. Confucianism, like Taoism, places importance on *chi* (energy). When a person's *chi* is debilitated and spent, the *yin* and *yang* spirits of the person separate and death occurs. Confucianism has a nonagitated attitude toward death.

NEO-CONFUCIANISM

Neo-Confucianism covers the developments in Confucianism from the Song Dynasty to the end of the Qing Age, 1644–1911 CE. Neo-Confucianism, like its predecessor, does not have any creeds or dogmas. It developed as a result of questions raised by the attractively presented Taoism and Buddhism. A number of schools of Neo-Confucianism developed combining the metaphysical elements of these teachings with traditional Confucian teaching, which included the need to investigate all aspects of "being." Such investigation is not merely to gain knowledge but to "rectify the mind." This also confirmed the teaching of Confucius that education was primarily for building character and self-cultivation.

The needs of Confucists and Neo-Confucists are similar and therefore are here treated together.

DIET

The Chinese approach to medicine and health is influenced by their doctrine of *chi* flowing harmoniously throughout the whole body. Illness is evidence that there is a disruption to the body's energy flow and energy levels. The holistic approach of Chinese philosophy is also applied to health. The mind is one element in the conditioning of bodily health, along with diet and food taken into the body. The responsibility for caring for health is a personal responsibility of which diet is an important part. Dietary needs of a Chinese patient, whether Confucian or Taoist, should be discovered so that the mind will be at rest over the nourishment that the body receives. The right diet will help restore the harmony of *chi* in the body.

AUTOPSIES, TRANSPLANTS, ORGAN DONATIONS

The veneration of ancestors applies to the way the dying or deceased person's body is handled in the health institution. To mutilate the body of a person in any way is considered to be sacrilegious and does not show respect for the body or the personhood of the deceased.

CHINESE BUDDHISM

The consensus is that Buddhism was introduced into China in 65 CE. Emperor Ming had a dream that resulted in the sending of emissaries to India who returned two years later with two Buddhist monks. The dream is reported to be about a golden man with a bright halo around his head. The first, native-born Chinese Buddhist monks were accepted officially in the fourth century.

Taoism and Buddhism, although having many

philosophical similarities, were in constant conflict with the favor of the emperor alternating between the two. In the ninth century, 4,500 Buddhist monasteries were destroyed and 265,000 monks and nuns forced to return to secular life. Chinese Buddhism has never fully regained its lost status.

Buddhism, however, has survived largely because Mahayana Buddhism has more to say about the life to come than Confucianism and Taoism, which are rather vague. Also, Buddhism has a more worldwide acceptance than the other two. In the twenty-first century, Taoism and Chinese Buddhism are better known outside China than they were a few decades earlier. There are a number of Chinese Buddhist schools established in Western countries, and temples of both can be found on all five continents. Taoism is also better known through its temples. It has gained some popularity through its martial arts and *Tai Chi.*

Venerable Master Hsing Yun has established his Hsi Lai University in California, and is typical of other Buddhist masters who seek to proclaim the message of universal happiness, the breaking down of generational differences and promoting harmony in community in the Mahayanan tradition.

➜ TEN ➜

Japanese Beliefs and Practices

For many in the Western world little is known of these people who, prior to World War II, remained largely within their own country and restricted entry by Westerners. Since its rapid economic growth and expansion, Japan is now a recognized world influence. Most people in Western countries are meeting Japanese people for the first time these days. They are welcomed as tourists and commercial investors.

There is still a basic ignorance of the Japanese and their culture, but the increasing possibility of Japanese people being admitted to our hospitals requires that some of that ignorance be overcome. However, the scope of this section permits only a very brief glimpse into the culture of the Japanese.

RELIGION IN JAPAN

When speaking of religion in Japan, we are thinking of many varieties. There is evidence that the Japanese are a very religious people. This was certainly the case up to World War II. The defeat of the Japanese in that war had repercussions upon the religion of the emperor, whose family claims direct descent from the sun goddess, Amaterasu. That the God-Emperor Hirohito could be defeated shook much religious belief. The postwar industrial development of Japan seems to have weakened the structure of the society on which religion largely depended. The practice of religion in Japan today is a minority pursuit; a recent survey shows 30 to 35 percent of adults with religious affiliations, yet 70 percent believe that religious sentiment is important.

The indigenous religion of Japan is Shintoism. This has been part of Japanese life for some two thousand years. Confucianism, which came to Japan via Korea during the sixth century CE, has often been considered more of a philosophy, with moral and ethical precepts, than a religion. About the same time Buddhism was introduced from China and rapidly gained royal patronage.

St. Francis Xavier introduced Christianity to Japan in 1549. It spread and grew quite rapidly; but the current Christian population is less than 1 percent.

The common people have amalgamated many religious practices to form syncretic folk religions, known as "new religious movements," some of which were established earlier but gained official recognition only after 1949. The new religions appeal to the people who are lost in the concrete jungles of urban living. They are strong in magical practice, with an emphasis on relevant issues such as family and health, and are not concerned with the religious questions on the future life. In this section, Shintoism and Japanese Buddhism will be expanded to further Westerners' understanding of their beliefs and practices.

SHINTOISM

The name *Shinto* goes back to prehistoric times. The religion has undergone much transformation from its earliest beginnings and has affected the sociocultural life of Japan's people. Even in the twentieth century, its political ramifications echoed around the world during World War II.

Currently it may be considered under four main forms: *Shinto* of the imperial house, shrine *Shinto*, sect *Shinto* and folk *Shinto*.

Shinto *of the Imperial House*

This form involved the rites and worship of imperial ancestors and is observed at special royal family shrines. The emperor usually officiates at these ceremonies, to which rites the general public is not admitted. Its fate in Japan suffered as a result of World War II and Emperor Hirohito's "abdicating" his divine powers in 1945. On this basis the new constitution of Japan was adopted.

From the Meija era of the mid-nineteenth century, state *Shinto* developed as a combination of *Shinto* of the imperial house and shrine *Shinto*. State *Shinto* became a government institution, with the priests as government servants. This remained the case until the end of World War II.

Shrine Shinto

Shrine *Shinto* was separated from the state in February 1946, becoming a purely religious body. The main principles of shrine *Shinto* are:

- To be grateful for the blessings of the *Kami* (the divine beings of heaven and earth) and the blessings of the ancestors, and to be diligent in the observance of *Shinto* rituals, applying oneself to them with sincerity, cheerfulness and purity of heart.

- To be helpful to others in the world at large through deeds of service, without thought of reward, and to seek the advancement of the world as one whose life mediates the will of the *Kami.*

- To bind oneself with others in harmonious acknowledgment of the will of the emperor, praying that the country may flourish and that other peoples too may live in peace and prosperity.

The shrines built as places of worship are to be plain in design and material, characterized by simplicity, purity and harmony. They house ashes and relics of the dead, store works of art, and are the dwelling places of the *Kami.*

Rituals principally are for purification, namely:

- *Rites of preliminary purification:* This involves the avoiding of all foods (except those prepared over a ritually pure fire) and the total immersion of the body in the sea or river. Certain taboos concerning recently bereaved persons and menstruating women are observed.

- *Rites of internal purification:* The priest, using a wand, symbolically cleanses the object or worshippers to be purified.
- *Rites of dedication:* Originating from harvest festival rituals, sprigs of the sacred sakaki tree, rice, sake, etc., are offered.

The prayers offering praise to the *Kami*, intercessions for blessing, personal dedication and pledges of right loving complete the service.

Successive generations are represented in the *Kami*, which place value on ancestors and the importance of future generations.

Sect Shinto

The promulgation of freedom of religion in Japan in 1889 created a problem for the government: The thirteen religious groups that sprang up between 1876 and 1908 were typical of *Shinto* forms, but the state was loathe to absorb them into shrine *Shinto*, so sect *Shinto*, which would embrace those groups, was adopted. Like the postwar new religions, sect *Shinto* emphasized contemporary life in contrast with stress upon any future life.

Folk Shinto

Folk *Shinto* is a primitive kind if Shintoism that is a mixture of superstition, magic religious rites, kinship ties and practices of the common people.

BUDDHISM

Buddhism was introduced into Japan about 538 CE, an early convert being Prince Shotoku about the year 600 CE, who saw Buddhism as a means of attaining his two goals:

- to establish a single central government under the authority of the emperor, thus unifying the various clans;
- to raise the cultural level of Japan.

Even at this period there were desires to keep Japanese values intact and to adapt Buddhism to fit these. A century later temples were being built with government subsidies. Some major developments of Buddhism took place:

- Appearing from China, whose culture was seen to be more advanced, Buddhism was embraced by the Japanese Imperial Family and the aristocracy, so it moved from aristocracy downward.

- The patronage of the emperor resulted in a strong bond between Buddhism and the state. This relationship is significantly unique. For instance, every citizen was to register at a particular temple.
- Buddhism adapted itself into the family life of Japan with a strong emphasis on ancestor worship and holding services for the dead.

FOLK RELIGION

Folk religion may include worship at family *Shinto* or Buddhist shrines as well as at village sites to honor the particular *Kami*. Ancestors are worshipped for their support in the practical things of life: the future, illness and similar matters. Weddings are usually performed according to *Shinto* tradition, while funerals are the prerogative of the Buddhist priests.

Many of the newer religions in Japan, such as sect *Shinto*, are traceable back to folk religion; the influence of folk religion stretches across all strata of society from urban to nonurban, the affluent to the poor.

NAMES

According to Japanese convention the family name comes first, then the given name. Some Japanese travelers and those who are living in Western countries are following the Western practice of putting the given name first, then the family name. It would be prudent to establish which is the family name to maintain true medical records and identification.

CARE OF THE ILL AND DYING

Informing patients and relatives of diagnosis

If the illness is neither terminal nor life-threatening then the doctor may inform the patient and family of all the facts. Many Japanese doctors do not tell their patients and patients do not ask.

Japanese culture involves subtle innuendo when the condition is terminal. Doctors hesitate to give any diagnosis and prognosis; they merely say that more tests which may require prolonged hospitalization are needed. When the condition has exhausted treatment possibilities, the specialist will suggest the patient may go home, indicating that the patient may go home to die in comfort and peace with the family. The family usually knows the truth, though Japanese people tend to believe that the patient may not be emotionally capable of handling the true diagnosis. The family then accepts the responsibility to emotionally support and comfort the terminal patient.

LENGTH OF HOSPITALIZATION

Japanese expect to spend longer periods in the hospital than is the case generally in the West. For a minor operation a week to ten days is normal, while for major surgery, it may be a month or more. This is partly due to health insurance schemes, where the longer the stay, the cheaper it becomes. There are three types:

- national insurance where government pays approximately 70 percent;
- company insurance where company pays approximately 90 percent;
- worker's compensation where insurance pays approximately 60 percent.

The length of stay in the hospital should be explained so that a Japanese patient does not consider the treatment not as adequate or good as in Japan.

DIET AND FASTING

Rice is the staple food of Japan, with very little spicy or fried content. Western hospital food is normally acceptable. The Japanese eat rice gruel (*Okayu*) when convalescing. (It is a simple one measure of rice to two of water slowly boiled until tender and soft, a little salt added during the cooking.) *Okayu* may be offered to the patient as the Japanese are reticent about making direct requests.

PASTORAL AND SPIRITUAL CARE

In Japanese Buddhism, prayer is important for personal benefits. In the Western world, the possibility of a *Shinto* or Japanese Buddhist priest being available is unlikely. A Japanese patient would not expect any form of pastoral or spiritual care, but the hospital chaplain may be able to provide spiritual support and be a religious presence to the patient. A short prayer by the chaplain using the name of God rather than Jesus would generally be accepted.

Should a suitable Buddhist priest or nun be available, it is, of course, advisable to seek the patient's permission to call him or her.

AUTOPSIES, TRANSFUSIONS, TRANSPLANTS

Japan is keen to catch up in the transplant field of medicine, though traditional ethics have largely been against transplants.

Live donor transplants of kidneys in Japan have taken place, although medical ethics committees are still debating the matter. Thus questions of transplants and organ donation at this stage would probably receive a negative response, although some Japanese opt for overseas transplant operations to avoid the Japanese bans and indecision.

Transfusions produce a clouded response; the AIDS situation may be a deterrent. A fear for the Japanese in a hospital outside of Japan is that "foreign" blood may be contaminated, thus creating a reluctance to accept a transfusion. Ascertain from relatives or patient the attitude to transfusions.

Autopsies for coroners' courts or to ascertain the exact cause of death are generally accepted. If a Japanese tourist should die, there is a possibility that an autopsy would be necessary if there is little previous medical history available.

ABLUTIONS

In Japan, the Japanese use Asian-type toilet facilities, that is, they require water for toilet cleansing purposes. In the West, they adapt readily to Western bathroom fixtures; most are comfortable using toilet paper. However, there may be a few who need water to be made available.

Water for washing hands before meals is another requirement.

MODESTY

Japanese women generally are very modest in matters concerning their body. They prefer to be treated by a nurse or doctor of the same sex. However, they recognize the professionalism of hospital personnel and are willing to waive this preference. Particular efforts should be made by male health workers to respect the dignity of Japanese women in their care.

Handling the deceased body

All jewelry is to be removed and returned to the family. Where family or priest's counsel is unavailable, normal procedure will be acceptable to the Japanese, who will later follow their own customs.

The Japanese would not expect foreigners to prepare a patient in Buddhist style; this becomes a family responsibility. Where the family is unavailable, a Buddhist priest should be notified if possible. The deceased is dressed in a white kimono and wears straw shoes called *waraji*. The ceremonial clothing is called *shiro shozoku*.

→ ELEVEN ←

Baha'i Faith

The Baha'i faith is the newest of the major independent religions of the world. It originated in Iran in the mid-nineteenth century. The founder was the prophet Baha'u'llah, which means "Glory to God."

The spread of this faith has been rather rapid. In 1984 it was reported as having over 112,000 centers and over 130 national bodies, and five years later the report added at least another 70 to the list of countries. Its followers come from almost every cultural, social, racial and religious background.

The prophet had an often difficult history, experiencing much persecution throughout his ministry. He was exiled to Akka (in modern Israel) where he died in 1892. He believed in God's progressive revelation to humankind, himself being the latest of the prophets.

Baha'i is an independent religion having its own laws and ordinances. It cannot be said to be a sect or reform movement of any other religion or philosophical system. Unity, concord and harmony remain the core of its philosophy.

The unity of God and his prophets and the human race is basic to Baha'ism, so it encompasses and accepts most religions. This belief in the value of life and equality within life leads to the promotion of equal opportunities for all; the respect for life stresses universal peace. Religion and science are also inseparable; through this union a peaceful, ordered and progressive community is possible.

Each person possesses a soul that moves into another life after death. Cultivation of this soul is possible through obligatory daily prayer and Scripture readings each morning and evening. Baha'i belief in the immortality of the soul generates a confidence that there will be a new and greater life in the hereafter.

DIET AND FASTING

Baha'i followers do not subscribe to any special dietary laws. Some may be vegetarians, though this is not a religious requirement. Baha'is do not drink alcohol except under medical direction.

Baha'is between the ages of fifteen and seventy are expected to fast between sunrise and sunset from March 2 to March 21 each year. However fasting is not compulsory during hospitalization, any illness, pregnancy; menstruation or when breast feeding.

RITUALS

There are no special religious requirements in cases of crisis. Birth is considered to be a happy occasion. Personal preference dictates the presence or otherwise of the husband at the time of delivery.

Ablutions and toilet practices demand no special requirements.

CARE OF THE ILL AND DYING

There is no priesthood and no sacramental requirements in the nursing or medical care of the sick. Therefore religious or pastoral care is of an entirely personal nature and is offered by religious friends or close relatives. The Baha'i writings contain many prayers and meditations for spiritual and physical healing. These offer comfort and guidance to the patient and to relatives and friends.

Handling of the deceased body

There are no specific religious rituals prior to or following death. Normal nursing procedures are acceptable. A deceased Baha'i may be wearing an inscribed ring, usually on the third or fourth finger of the right hand. This should not be buried with the body. The ring and any Baha'i books should be kept aside and given into the care of Baha'i relatives or members of the Baha'i community. The handing over of these things to a Baha'i is important if the deceased's relatives do not share the faith.

Under normal circumstances cremation is not allowed. The body must be buried within one hour's distance of the place of death. The burial service consists of Baha'i prayers and readings from sacred texts. Recognized funeral directors may be used.

AUTOPSIES, TRANSFUSIONS, TRANSPLANTS

These are acceptable if performed on sound medical advice.

An autopsy is acceptable as long as the body is treated and returned with dignity.

A Baha'i may leave his or her body for medical research on the proviso that the body is buried with dignity and not cremated or otherwise disposed of.

Organ donations are equally acceptable on similar conditions, that dignity is maintained. The donation of organs is in line with the Baha'i philosophy of helping other people and of ensuring harmony in the world.

ABORTION AND
FAMILY PLANNING

The soul comes into being at conception. Abortion is therefore strongly discouraged, except for legitimate medical reasons, on the advice of a physician or preferably a panel of doctors.

Contraception presents no conflict for the Baha'i. However, in vitro fertilization or other artificial means of conception are considered improper.

MODESTY

Baha'is generally have no preference for female or male health-care professionals during their hospitalization. Their belief in the unity of science and religion gives them a great respect for medical personnel and medical advice, which leads to a belief that prescribed medications and prayer combine in the healing process.

✦ APPENDIX ✦

Religious Food Observance

The observance of food law is an important part of some traditions. To break a food law would be unthinkable; some would be physically repulsed. Guilt, disgust, shame and even illness sometimes ensue when even inadvertently one of these laws is infringed.

Westernization has weakened the resolve of many to maintain religious food prescriptions. Patients' dietary needs should be part of the questionnaire at the time of hospital admission so that the patient's requirements can be accommodated.

Guidelines:
Permitted and Prohibited Foods

	Hindus Buddhists	Sikhs	Muslims	Jews
Eggs	some*	yes	yes	yes
Milk and yogurt	yes	yes	yes	yes
Cottage/ curd cheese	yes	yes	yes	yes
Chicken	some*	some	*halal*[+]	kosher[++]
Mutton	some*	some	*halal*[+]	kosher[++]
Beef	no	no	*halal*[+]	kosher[++]
Pork	no	rarely	no	no
Fish	some*	some	yes	yes
Butter/*ghee*	yes	yes	yes	yes
Margarine/ vegetable oils	yes	yes	yes	yes

* Very strict followers avoid this.

[+] *Halal* meat must be killed, dedicated and prepared in a special way.

[++] Kosher meat for Jews requires special rituals and butchering procedures in preparation.

→ REFERENCES ←

Agency for Cultural Affairs. *Japanese Religion: A Survey.* 7th edition. Tokyo: Kodansha, 1989.

Carmody, Denise Lardner, and John Tully Carmody. *Prayer in World Religions.* Maryknoll, N.Y.: Orbis, 1990.

Fisher, Mary Pat. *Living Religious.* 2nd edition. Englewood Cliffs, Colo.: Prentice Hall, 1994.

Hospital Chaplaincies Council. *Our Ministry and Other Faiths.* London: C 10 Publications, 1983.

Kirkwood, Neville A. *Pastoral Care to Muslims.* New York: Haworth, 2002.

Lothian Community Relations Council. *Religions and Cultures: A Guide to Patient Belief.* Edinburgh: Lothian Community Relations Council, 1984.

Neuberger, Julia. *Caring for Dying People of Different Faiths*. London: Austen Cornish Publishers, 1987.

Nursing Times. "Death with Dignity" series, vol. 85. London, 1989.

Windish, Paul. *Thorsons Principles of Taoism*. London: HarperCollins, 2000.